Healthy City Projects in Developing Countries

An International Approach to Local Problems

Edmundo Werna, Trudy Harpham,
Ilona Blue and Greg Goldstein

EARTHSCAN
Earthscan Publications Ltd, London

First published in the UK in 1998 by
Earthscan Publications Ltd

Copyright © Edmundo Werna, Trudy Harpham, Ilona Blue and Greg Goldstein, 1998

All rights reserved

A catalogue record for this book is available from the British Library

ISBN: 1 85383 455 6 (paperback)
ISBN: 1 85383 456 4 (hardback)

Typesetting by JS Typesetting, Wellingborough, Northants

Printed and bound by Biddles Ltd, Guildford and King's Lynn

Cover design by Declan Buckley
Cover photograph © Sean Sprague, Panos Pictures

For a full list of publications, please contact
Earthscan Publications Ltd
120 Pentonville Road
London N1 9JN
Tel: 0171 278 0433
Fax: 0171 278 1142
email:earthinfo@earthscan.co.uk
http://www.earthscan.co.uk

Earthscan is an editorially independent subsidiary of Kogan Page Ltd and publishes in association with WWF-UK and the International Institute for Environment and Development.

This book is printed on elemental chlorine free paper from sustainably managed forests.

Contents

Preface iv
About the Authors vi
List of Acronyms and Abbreviations viii
List of Illustrations x

Chapter 1   Introduction 1

Chapter 2   Establishing Healthy City Projects 21

Chapter 3   Implementing Healthy City Projects 52

Chapter 4   Evaluating Healthy City Projects 86

Chapter 5   Are Healthy Cities Sustainable? 104

Chapter 6   Conclusion 122

References 135

Index 144

Preface

Interest in the theme of this book originated from our professional experience in establishing, implementing and evaluating healthy city projects in developing countries. Three of the authors (Edmundo, Trudy and Ilona) have worked as consultants for the WHO (World Health Organization) in such activities. Greg, in his turn, is the Global Co-ordinator for the Healthy City Project at the WHO headquarters. We all thank the WHO for its support of our work in healthy cities, which enabled us to produce the raw material for this book. Also, the WHO has received funds from the DGIS (Dutch Bilateral Aid Agency) to sponsor a great part of the consultancy work of Edmundo, Trudy and Ilona. Therefore, DGIS's contribution is also appreciated.

Parts of three chapters of this book include adaptations of material taken from articles and a book chapter previously written by two of us. Chapter 2 was adapted from Werna and Harpham's 'The Implementation of the Healthy Cities Project' (published in *Habitat International* (1996) 20(2), pp221–228). Chapter 4 was adapted from Werna and Harpham's 'The Evaluation of the Healthy Cities Project in Developing Countries' (published in *Habitat International* (1995) 19(4), pp629–641). Finally, Chapter 5 was adapted from Harpham and Werna's 'Sustainability in Urban Health' (published in *Habitat International* (1996) 20(3), pp421–429), and from Harpham and Werna's 'Healthy Cities and its Application' (published in Pugh, C (ed) (1996) *Sustainability, the Environment and Urbanization* Earthscan, London, pp63–81). Therefore, the editors and publishers of these sources also have our gratitude.

We would also like to take the opportunity to thank many other people who have been involved in healthy city projects, in the field

Preface

and at the WHO headquarters and regional offices, from whom we learned a great deal. It is not possible to mention everyone individually here, but they all have our deepest gratitude.

In addition to the collective acknowledgements made above, we have important individual notes. Edmundo's share of the writing up of this book was carried out at the Department of Civil Construction Engineering of the University of São Paulo. Therefore, the support given by this Department is kindly acknowledged, with special thanks to Professor Alex Abiko and Professor Vahan Agopyan. On a personal note, Edmundo appreciates the kaleidoscopic support given by Liliana Ishihata, to whom he dedicates his work in this book. Finally, given that this is a book about health, Edmundo would like to pay homage to the late Paulo Ernesto Salvo, who inspired him with his contagious joy of living – perhaps the best indicator of health. Trudy and Ilona's share of the writing up of this book was carried out at the School of Urban Development and Policy of the South Bank University where the final editing of the manuscript took place. We are grateful for the administrative support provided. Finally, Greg, a member of the WHO's staff, thanks the Organization for supporting his writing up time.

Edmundo Werna, Trudy Harpham, Ilona Blue and Greg Goldstein
Sao Paulo, London and Geneva
February 1998

About the Authors

Edmundo Werna is the Urban Adviser to the United Nations Volunteer Programme. He previously worked in Brazil and the UK as a researcher and consultant on urban development in developing countries with a particular focus on urban management, the environment and health. He has published several articles in academic and technical journals, written two books and co-edited *Urban Health Research: Implications for Policy* (1996 CAB International, UK).

Trudy Harpham is Professor of Urban Development and Policy at South Bank University, London. Previously, she headed the Urban Health Programme of the London School of Hygiene and Tropical Medicine (1990–1995). Her research interests include: the impact of urbanization on health (both mental and physical); the links between health services and environmental health; and the re-evaluation of city-wide health master planning. She has written extensively on urban health in developing countries and has co-edited three books including the widely cited *In the Shadow of the City: Community Health and the Urban Poor* (1988 Oxford University Press, Oxford).

Ilona Blue is a Research Fellow in urban health working at the School of Urban Development and Policy, South Bank University, London. She was previously a Research Assistant on the Urban Health Programme at the London School of Hygiene and Tropical Medicine. Her research interests include intra-urban differentials in health, mental health, and linking social and health agendas. She has published a number of articles on urban health issues and she co-edited the book *Urbanization and Mental Health in Developing Countries* with Trudy Harpham.

About the Authors

Greg Goldstein has worked in the Urban Environmental Health Unit in the World Health Organization Programme on Environmental Health, Geneva for the last ten years. He is Co-ordinator for Healthy Cities (Asia, Africa, Latin America). Particular areas of work and interest include: urban health development and city health planning; the development and application of indicators on health and environment; social marginalization of peri-urban dwellers; and health issues of small-scale industries (SSIs). He has assisted in the development of local solutions to health and environment issues and has published guidance manuals for healthy cities work. For ten years prior to joining the WHO he was a lecturer in the Department of Public Health, University of Sydney, working with students from Australia and many Asian and Pacific countries on MPH (Masters in Public Health) or related degree courses. He worked as Project Manager for the Pakistan Health Financing Study, 1986–1987.

List of Acronyms and Abbreviations

ADAB	Association of Development Agencies of Bangladesh
ADP	annual development programme
BMA	Bangkok Metropolitan Administration
CBO	community-based organization
DALY	disability-adjusted life year
DFID	Department for International Development (UK)
DGIS	Dutch Bilateral Aid Agency (translation)
GIS	geographical information systems
HEADLAMP	Health and Environment Analysis for Decision-making – Linkage Analysis and Monitoring Project (WHO)
ICLEI	International Council for Local Environmental Initiatives
ILO	International Labour Office
IULA	International Union of Local Authorities
LIFE	Local Initiative for the Environment (UNDP)
MoH	Ministry of Health
MCAP	multi-city action plan
MPH	Masters in Public Health
NGO	non-governmental organization
ODA	Overseas Development Administration (UK)
PAHO	Pan-American Health Organization
QDA	Quetta Development Authority
QMC	Quetta Municipal Corporation
SSI	Cottage and small-scale industry
UN	United Nations
UNCED	United Nations Conference on Environment and Development

List of Acronyms and Abbreviations

UNCHS	United Nations Centre for Human Settlements
UNDP	United Nations Development Programme
UNEP	United Nations Environment Programme
UNESCO	United Nations Education, Science and Culture Organization
UNICEF	United Nations Children's Fund
USAID	United States Agency for International Development
WHO	World Health Organization

List of Illustrations

Chapter 1
Box	1.1	Principles of Health for All	5
Box	1.2	Definition of Environmental Health	13
Box	1.3	Why Settings Are Important	17
Box	1.4	Core Healthy City Concepts	18

Chapter 2
Box	2.1	The Steering Committee of the Chittagong Healthy City Project	23
Box	2.2	Outline of a Municipal Health Plan	28
Table	2.1	A 'Snapshot' of the Chittagong Health Plan: Part of the Plan of Action of the Water and Sewerage Task Force	30
Box	2.3	The Hand of Central Government in Chittagong	38

Chapter 3
Box	3.1	Ten Questions around which Information can be Organized	56
Table	3.1	Qualitative and Quantitative Methods	65
Box	3.2	Priority Areas in Fayoum, Egypt	78
Box	3.3	Initial List of Priorities for Quetta Healthy City Project	80
Box	3.4	Examples of Healthy City Project Activities	84

Chapter 4
Table	4.1	Selected Indicators for Evaluation of Healthy City Projects	94
Box	4.1	The Qualities of a Healthy City	102

List of Illustrations

Chapter 5
Table 5.1 Actors Involved in the Chittagong Healthy City Project — 115
Figure 5.1 The Actors in Bangkok Healthy City Project — 117
Figure 5.2 Twenty Steps for Developing a Healthy City Project of Bangkok Metropolitan Administration — 118

1 Introduction

THE OBJECTIVES OF THIS BOOK

The 'healthy city' initiative, which began in 1987 with World Health Organization (WHO) support, is a development activity that seeks to put health on the agenda of decision makers in cities, to build a strong lobby for public health at the local level, and to develop a local, participatory approach to dealing with health and environmental problems. Ultimately, the initiative aims to improve the physical, mental, social and environmental well-being of the people who live and work in urban areas.

Most experience of healthy city projects has been in industrialized countries. However, there is a growing number of initiatives in developing countries and increasing interest from the international community about the nature and direction of healthy cities in the developing world. This interest has been heightened by: the 1996 United Nations (UN) summit on cities which emphasized action at the local, urban government (municipal) level; the focus of the 1996 World Health Day on healthy cities; and the increased poverty focus of many bilateral and multilateral aid agencies (for example, the UK's Department for International Development (DFID), formerly the Overseas Development Administration (ODA)). In response to such interest this book aims to:

- describe the different phases of healthy city projects including planning, implementation and evaluation;
- illustrate the above phases with examples of healthy city projects in developing countries;

- consider the sustainability of healthy city projects; and
- draw together existing knowledge of healthy city projects in developing countries and provide some guidance for their future development.

The intended audience includes urban development practitioners with an interest in health, the international health community (both academics and policy makers), and those involved with healthy cities in both industrialized and developing countries.

This first chapter sets the scene by considering the amount of interest in health in cities of the developing world, emphasizing the importance of intersectoral action, and highlighting those trends in urban development which have implications for health.

HEALTH IN CITIES: IS IT IMPORTANT?

This is a book about public health in cities, and herein lies a problem. This subject is bedevilled with a profound lack of interest. Attention is given to urban conditions, it must be granted, when gridlock causes paralysis of traffic; when people are advised to stay indoors because the air is unsafe to breathe; when the level of violence crosses various thresholds. But in general, complacency is the order of the day.

It is not obvious why this is so. More and more people live in cities. The proportion of the world's population living in cities is over 45 per cent and rising, while in 1900 it was only 14 per cent. This 'urbanization' is perhaps the biggest social change in the history of mankind. Around the world people in cities face escalating urban problems. For one third or even half of the inhabitants of a given city, there may be poverty; insufficient food; crowded, makeshift housing; insecure tenure; poor waste disposal; and unsafe working conditions. These living conditions cause health problems, ranging from communicable diseases and malnutrition to mental illnesses and chronic respiratory diseases. Every type of human misery from crime to drugs to epidemic disease finds fertile soil in squatter settlements and peri-urban fringes. But strangely, the poverty and

Introduction

vulnerability represented by the world's cities are tolerated and even exploited. Such conditions are accepted almost as naturally ordained.

While a majority of the cities of the world face crumbling infrastructure, declining services and a looming water shortage, scientific and technological advances have become so routine they fail to excite and inspire. A connection between advanced technology and scientific capacity to improve the living conditions in cities and of their poor citizens is never made. A Spanish colleague who marvels at the wonders of science suspects humankind must be under a curse to permit such settlements and asks 'Why then don't we live with more dignity?' An Indian politician chastens us for expecting things to be different: 'progress is not inherent in history – it is an English concept, and a failed concept'.*

This is not the position taken in this book. The book is dedicated to change and progress. It is a book about a public health programme called the Healthy City Project also known as the healthy city approach, or sometimes the healthy city movement. This flexibility of terms is maintained in this book. Some cities have decided to name their healthy city activities a 'project' while others have used the term 'programme'.

This chapter will show that the Healthy City Project has adopted ideas from many sources. It has incorporated the hard-earned wisdom of the 'sanitary idea' of England, of the Alma Ata Conference (on) primary health care, of the Ottawa Charter for Health Promotion, the Rio Conference on Environment and Development and its Agenda 21, and more recently of Habitat II (the City Summit) and the habitat agenda.

The WHO Healthy City programme is a public health approach that builds upon the time-honoured idea that living and environmental conditions are responsible for health. Cities have to deal with health problems arising from many people living and working

---

* The comments by the 'Spanish colleague' and the 'Indian politician' have been taken from a report by Flora Lewis of a UNESCO Conference in Valencia in January 1997 ('Challenges of the Third Millennium' *International Herald Tribune* 31 January 1997).

together in close proximity. 'The ancient Greeks regarded illness as a disturbance of the natural balance between the internal and external environments of the person, while the Romans made a contribution to public health through the provision of good water supplies, roads and housing' (Davies and Kelly 1993: p1). McKeown found that – contrary to popular belief – the major factor in the improvement in health in the UK and other developed countries in the 19th and 20th centuries was not advances in medical care and technology, but certain social, environmental and economic changes (WHO 1995a):

- limitation of family size;
- increase in food supplies;
- a healthier physical environment; and
- specific preventive and therapeutic measures.

One may trace three important strands in the development of healthy city projects: Ottawa Charter, 'new public health' and Health Promotion; Alma Ata, urban primary health care and the district health system; and the emergence of local government as a major development force and key player in health and environment since 1992.

Ottawa Charter

The Ottawa Charter has made a substantial contribution to the development of the more holistic approach needed to develop physical, social and economic environments, which better promote and maintain the health of populations. The Charter enunciated five action areas to improve health: building healthy public policy; creating supportive environments; strengthening community action; developing personal skills; and reorienting health services (WHO 1986). Following the development of the Ottawa Charter in 1985, the European office of the WHO proposed a health promotion project to be known as the Healthy City Project. The idea was to demonstrate the Ottawa Charter in action, 'taking Health for All strategy off the shelves and into the streets of European cities' (Ashton and Seymour 1988). The intention of the Project was to devise ways to apply the principles and strategies of Health for All described below through local action in cities and to put it on the agenda of local government. Initially, 11 European cities agreed to participate in a healthy city project that would address health issues across sectors such as education, housing, transport, community services, and in planning. The healthy city idea spread rapidly beyond the limits of the initial project to cities and towns across Europe, and it has been influential in the development of healthy city projects in other regions of the world.

Alma Ata, Urban Primary Health Care and the District Health System

The WHO, from its beginning in 1946, has long recognized the interaction of physical, mental and social factors in determining health. In 1978, the WHO launched a major public health movement called 'Health for All' at Alma Ata, based on six principles that reflect McKeown's concern that social, environmental and economic factors in health receive due attention (see Box 1.1).

Box 1.1 Principles of Health for All

- Reduced inequalities in health
- Emphasis on prevention of diseases
- Intersectoral co-operation including reducing environmental risks
- Community participation
- Emphasis on primary health care in health care systems
- International co-operation

The basic concepts and components of primary health care have had a major influence on health systems around the world, and primary health care has been described as the key to achieving health for all. During the 1970s and 1980s the main emphasis in community health in developing countries was on extending health service coverage in rural areas, but since then urban health problems have been highlighted (Rossi-Espagnet et al 1991). While health facilities and services are more concentrated in urban areas as compared to rural areas, poor urban neighbourhoods receive low priority and may be highly disadvantaged, at the same time experiencing serious health risks and high morbidity due to crowded and unsanitary living conditions. An urban district no less than a rural district may be a focus for a comprehensive district health system that includes access to primary and higher levels of health care, and preventive health services and activities.

The Healthy City programme has defined an important role for the health sector in relation to improving living conditions and addressing environment issues in urban development. It is based on the mandate of health authorities to set health goals and targets, and their access to health status (and disease causation) information, and the necessary analytical capability. In many countries the role of environmental health units within the Ministry of Health is changing in a way that may facilitate health inputs into development planning. Many countries are transferring the traditional Ministry of Health responsibilities for provision of various environmental services, such as water and sanitation services, solid waste management, or environmental health inspection of food markets or restaurants to other ministries or departments. The change moves the emphasis away from environmental health *services*, towards health information, monitoring and analysis, health policy development, and health promotion and advocacy. In a number of countries the health sector is now active in initiating healthy city programmes.

Emergence of Local Government as a Major Development Force and Key Player in Health and Environment since 1992

The United Nations Conference on Environment and Development (UNCED) held in Rio de Janeiro in 1992, and its global action plan Agenda 21, served to raise awareness and focus attention on global issues of environment and development. The Conference demonstrated the need for a development model that preserves environmental resources and ecosystems for the benefit of future generations. Agenda 21 specifically noted that the wellbeing of humans was 'at the centre of concerns for sustainable development'. The Rio Conference also underlined the importance of local action and community participation in development, and served to place local government firmly on the development agenda. This theme was taken up in development conferences throughout the decade, and full recognition of the major role of local government and of 'participatory local governance' was apparent at the Habitat II Conference in Istanbul in 1996. National plans to implement Agenda 21, and 'Local Agenda 21' plans that support sustainable development have provided an excellent context for healthy city work at both the national and local levels in many countries.

While the WHO has been identified with much of the above, one must keep in mind the Healthy City is both a specific programme of the WHO, and a less formal movement involving networks of cities within countries and regions in all parts of the world. The Healthy City Project has roots in the public health culture of many parts of the world, such as the local health systems in Latin America, the Health-Culture movement in Japan, and the urban planning traditions and practice of virtually all cultures.

Healthy city is an idea that has caught fire. In a few short years over 1,000 cities have adopted this approach to solving urban problems. But the coverage of the world's cities remains slight. What is needed is a major international effort to develop our towns and cities in such a way that all citizens can live a decent life – using existing capabilities and technologies.

As already mentioned there is a problem with a book about public health in cities, namely a lack of interest in the subject. Unfortunately there is another problem. There is nothing new in this book, that has not been written about extensively over the last decade. Nor is there in it a fundamental idea about public health that does not have clear lineage to public health writings of earlier decades and even centuries. Ashton (1992) in describing the evolution of public health in England demonstrated how the Health of Towns Association developed and advocated the sanitary idea of public health and achieved its enactment in legislation – the Public Health Act of 1848. The English sanitary idea has major elements of the current Healthy City programme, and can be summarized as:

- the legitimacy of working locally;
- resourcefulness and pragmatism;
- humanitarianism and a strong moral tone;
- the recognition of the need for special skills and qualifications;
- appropriate research and inquiry;
- the need to focus on 'positive' health (that is, to recognize that a programme to improve health may have a different emphasis to one that aims to control diseases, even if both have much in common);
- the value of producing reports on the state of health of the population;
- populism and 'health advocacy', and what is now called an 'intersectoral approach'; and
- the recognition that public health needs to be the responsibility of a democratically accountable body.

One may ask what was missing from the sanitary idea of the 1840s that is now within the healthy city approach? In terms of fundamentals, the answer is not much. One might complain about a lack of environmental sensibility, of discussion of the city as an ecosystem, or the absence of any idea of responsibility for stewardship of the environment for the benefit of future generations. Perhaps this is the price you pay when you are 150 years ahead of your time.

Why then was the sanitary idea lost? Ashton (1992) suggested that the germ theory of disease superseded the sanitary idea at the end of the 19th century, and paved the way for the development of vaccination, and subsequently the therapeutic era of public health commencing in the 1930s. Public health became dominated by the idea that diseases could be controlled by treatment and the implicit assumption that magic bullets could be provided by the pharmaceutical industry for all conditions. So powerful was this idea that to this day public health departments and leaders around the world focus on hospitals and clinics for treatment of the sick and wounded, and generally fail to make purposeful efforts to alter the social and living conditions that cause diseases and injuries.

The current challenges – one might say crises – affecting public health will now be briefly reviewed, as a prelude to introducing and explaining the nature of the Healthy City Project. A central focus of the discussion is 'intersectoral action', which, as we have seen, is not a new issue.

NEW CHALLENGES FOR PUBLIC HEALTH: THE OLD ISSUE OF 'INTERSECTORAL ACTION'

Current trends in health problems and patterns point to the need for intersectoral action. Throughout the world there are many unresolved health crises and problems, including diseases associated with poor housing and living conditions, new and re-emerging diseases, social health issues including violence, and mental ill health. Additional new challenges for public health include increased longevity in many regions, and more elderly people. There are new infectious diseases such as ebola, legionella and hanta virus, and many communicable diseases are resurgent, including dengue, cholera and plague. There have been rapid developments in communications and information technologies that can assist education – or can have the effect of eroding traditional lifestyles and promoting new lifestyles. Whilst age-old public health hazards such as unsafe food and water, microbiological contamination of the environment, overall poor sanitation and inadequate environmental hygiene are still prevalent, new environment and development problems have emerged, some of which, like climate change, appear to threaten the entire ecosystem (Editorial 1991; Editorial 1992; Epstein 1992; Kilburn 1995).

In both urban and rural areas worldwide, efforts to combat poverty and improve living standards have involved the development of industry (including cottage and small-scale industries (SSIs)) and/or intensification of agricultural production. Whilst these efforts have brought considerable benefits, they have also resulted in environmental problems such as pollution, chemical contamination and physical hazards in both settlements and workplaces. Occupational hazards are now as important in low income countries as they are in economically developed countries.

In this book the terms intersectoral collaboration, or using an 'integrated approach', will refer to any effort to ensure health issues are addressed in municipal and national plans and activities, by many key development sectors (industry, housing, local government, agriculture, transport, etc) (WHO 1992).

Intersectoral collaboration is listed as an element of primary health care, but out of all of the elements of primary health care, it may be the least successful (Tarimo and Webster 1994). Although intersectoral action has been an essential part of the WHO's Primary Health Care policy – especially since 1978 and the Alma Ata Conference – a report to the UN Commission on Sustainable Development in 1994, by the WHO (as Task Manager of Chapter 6 of Agenda 21), indicated that health issues are frequently *not* being addressed in many countries through development planning in key sectors. This apparent failure of intersectoral action is surprising, given the importance that a majority of health planners attach to it. One reason is the pervasive myth that good health is the result of medical and hospital services. There is a general lack of understanding of the nature of health, and specifically of the important influence of social and living conditions on health, sometimes by people within the health sector itself.

However there may be a second major reason for the failure of intersectoral action. As health sector workers, we have often blamed the housing sector, or the industry sector or local government, for ignoring health considerations in their work. We may have overlooked a problem within the health sector itself. The health sector at present in most countries is generally lacking the capacity to undertake studies or to collect data to measure or estimate the health impacts of development activities. It is arguable that until it develops

Introduction

this capacity, its ability to participate in intersectoral work may be limited. Health concerns and information, for example mortality and morbidity data, is of interest to other development sectors, only to the extent that:

■ some linkage can be established between the health problem being measured and the activities of the development sector. That is, the 'health burden' of the development activities should be measured (in terms of death, disability, etc), with an estimation of the contribution that the various social and environmental factors are making to health problems (for further details see Chapter 3); and
■ there is identification made, and promotion given to various 'health opportunities' presented by development programmes.

Thus urban development activities such as housing or industrial development have the potential to enhance the health status of the population *if* health promotion and protection measures are undertaken in implementing the development. For example, in industrial development, occupational safety considerations and pollution control should be integral, or in housing development, basic environmental services and primary health care measures should be implemented with community participation.

In addressing urban problems, a healthy city project does not seek to take over the management of the above functions from the competent authorities and agencies. Rather, it adds the health dimension to them by measurement of the health burden such problems create (in terms of death, disability, etc), and makes health issues relevant and understandable to the work of local government agencies and non-governmental agencies.

In most countries lack of attention to health in settlements planning and management has resulted in a down-stream role for the health sector, whereby it deals with the diseases and injuries caused by unhealthy living conditions, while lacking a significant capacity to change them. We shall see that the healthy city approach uses the construction of a city health plan as a framework for establishing a linkage between living conditions and health, and the subsequent efforts to improve living conditions.

It is now apparent that the health sector has paid too little attention to the living conditions in rural and urban settlements, which are of primary importance for influencing the level of health in any community. It is known that overall improvements in mortality and morbidity have generally come from higher standards of living and technological progress, rather than from regulation of building standards (Lotti 1991).

The Healthy City programme deals with all aspects of living conditions and their impact on health, including the physical environment, and social and economic conditions. To focus for a moment on the environment: it is clear that environmental considerations in urban planning and management require far greater attention. As well as negative health and social impacts, their neglect may impair urban productivity and restrict future development options, because of unsustainable use or damage to natural resources.

The limitations of conventional approaches to environmental health will be highlighted here to explain the emphasis in a healthy city project on building broad political support. It is evident that the challenges inherent in the area of health and environment today have become so complex and diverse that the health sector has found itself increasingly unable to define coherently its responsibilities in this area. The result has been that the public health basis of environmental management is being gradually eroded. Typical urban health and environment problems require government action and involve decisions on allocation of scarce resources. They nearly always require intersectoral action for health. They involve issues of equity, with citizens, industry, government agencies, scientists and others having an interest in the outcome of the policy implementation process. Walker (1994) in discussing environmental policy noted 'it is not merely a question of ecological and health risk assessment or cost benefit analysis but a range of issues including environmental monitoring and surveillance and the integration of programs, services and research into a unified cohesive framework'.

Box 1.2 Definition of Environmental Health

> The term environmental health is not used here in the traditional sense of provision of services for environmental hygiene, sanitary engineering, inspection, monitoring and control, but to also encompass efforts to improve living conditions (physical and social conditions) through attention to health considerations in the planning and management of rural and urban settlements.
>
> Source: WHO (1995a: p5)

However, current practice in public health may be unable to meet this new challenge where it is restricted to the provision of clinical services, and in the area of environmental health, limited to environmental hygiene, sanitary engineering, inspection, monitoring and control. Wide-ranging reforms are needed in order that the health sector may deal with the assessment and management of health risks in a framework of sustainable development. An increased emphasis on qualitative research, showing how the physical and social environment influences the quality of people's daily lives, is also needed (Editorial 1996).

Unfortunately there is a worldwide trend for the health sector to abdicate much of its responsibility for health and environment. At a time when health and environment issues are receiving more attention than they have in the past, it is ironic that the health sector has been slow to embrace the development of this 'Cinderella' discipline (Doll 1992). This has also contributed to deficits in properly trained environmental health personnel (Gordon 1990).

Attention to health and environment has been conspicuous by its absence in a number of key public health reports, such as the national 'Healthy People 2000' report in the US, and the inadequate representation of health and environment issues as reflected in the priorities of the American Public Health Association, where one finds an overemphasis on personal health and health care issues (Gordon 1992). Professionals not trained in environmental health exert greater influence on health and environment policy and priorities than the public health community.

Environmental health straddles the disciplines of environment and health and does not fall into the mainstream activities of either sector. Thus, neither sector has taken clear responsibility for it. Environmental health is intrinsically part of environmental management, in which many development sectors and agencies have important roles to play. It is also an intrinsic part of public health. Advocacy is needed to raise the profile and image of environmental health. In most countries, environmental health is relatively invisible, and is noticed only when things go drastically wrong. In addition, environmental health is often considered costly, and its benefits in terms of cases of disease that are prevented may be overlooked.

CHANGING HEALTH AND URBAN DEVELOPMENT PERSPECTIVES

Three new perspectives – discussed in UN conferences from Rio '92 (the Earth Summit) to Istanbul 1996 (Habitat II or the City Summit) – are changing public health, and have supported the emergence of the healthy city approach:

- The notion that health should be an integral component of settlements management and development, given that environmental exposures occur in places where people live and work (Editorial 1996; UNCHS 1996).
- The principle that health can be improved by modification of the physical environment, and social and economic conditions that affect health. The home, school, workplace, village and city are the places where people live, work and recreate (WHO 1996a; McDonald et al 1994).
- The change in emphasis in urban development and management, *away* from what national governments do in cities, *to* how national and provincial governments should support the efforts and initiatives of city and local governments, and those living and working in cities, including individual households, community organizations, non-governmental organizations (NGOs) and private sector institutions (World Resources Institute 1996).

Introduction

In relation to the third point: the question is *not* whether local action plays a greater role in the determination of living conditions than do national policies and programmes. Clearly it is vital to ensure that health issues are addressed in all development activities *both* at the national and local level. The point here is that the contribution of cities, towns and villages to the creation of housing, employment, education and other development work is both substantial and (in the past) relatively overlooked in development planning and management.

The role of local government is changing in response to the current challenges of municipal planning and management, and service provision, associated with rapid urbanization and urban population growth. A partnership model of service provision is emerging with services provided through the co-ordinated efforts of service users, local authorities and their affiliated service departments, private investors, local businesses, trade unions, religious groups, community organizations, central and provincial governments, and even international development and financial institutions. Co-ordination and management of local and municipal planning must engage and balance the interests of all these stakeholders and may best be carried out in a more decentralized manner at the level of local government, with national and provincial agencies playing a policy and support role. Typical objectives of local partnerships of stakeholders in city planning are:

- to create a shared community vision of the future;
- to identify and prioritize key issues;
- to raise awareness and facilitate community-based analysis of local issues;
- to develop action plans, drawing on the experiences and innovations of diverse local groups;
- to mobilize community-wide resources to meet service needs; and
- to increase public support for municipal programmes.

Local authorities have a particularly critical role in development, not only in investment, planning and management but also in encouraging and supporting the initiatives and innovations of the other groups within their city. An impressive aspect of Habitat II was the interest shown by local authorities in health and environment issues. This was not confined to statements in the Habitat II Agenda or the WHO-organized meetings at the conference, but was also evident in many health-related events that took place during the conference that were initiated by various local authorities.

We shall now focus on the contribution of the field of health promotion and in particular the role of advocacy and the 'settings' approach in healthy city work.

ROLE OF SETTINGS, ADVOCACY AND SOCIAL MOBILIZATION IN INTERSECTORAL COLLABORATION

Intersectoral action may be easier to achieve and more effective at local and municipal levels than at national level. The use of healthy settings (neighbourhoods, workplaces, cities, villages, health facilities, food markets, etc) facilitates people's participation and co-operation among development agencies and organizations. A local government health plan (for example, a city health plan, a neighbourhood health plan) is an appropriate mechanism for co-operation and for addressing health issues in a way that attracts community participation and also inputs from non-health professionals.

The settings approach has turned out to be a powerful and valuable one for the promotion of health in many countries (Mullen et al 1995). Health status is determined more by the living conditions in settings such as the above than by the health care facilities that are provided. Settings are major social structures that provide channels and mechanisms of influence for reaching defined populations. Each setting has a unique set of members, authorities, rules and participating organizations. Generally these structures are organized for more deeply binding purposes than the single mission of health. Mullen et al (1995) have described how the frequent interaction and patterns of membership and communication associated with settings create a good opportunity for social influence and health education (see Box 1.3).

Box 1.3 Why settings are important

- Provide channels for delivering health promotion programmes
- Diffusion of information is facilitated
- Represent relationships between participants, authorities and organizations
- Provide access to gatekeepers
- Provide entry points and access to specific populations
- Provide role for professionals

Source: Modified from Mullen et al (1995)

The Healthy City Project advocates the settings approach and emphasizes intersectoral collaboration at the local level. In healthy cities, there is a need for broad political support that encourages all key agencies to be involved and co-operate. Mayors and municipalities may commit themselves to a healthy city process, that involves formulating and adopting a 'Municipal Health Plan'. This involves work by many different agencies to prepare the plan. Developing solutions to problems on a community-wide basis requires partnerships between municipal government agencies (health, water, sanitation, housing, social welfare, etc), universities, NGOs, private companies, and community organizations and groups.

Health advocacy is needed to put health on the agenda of decision makers, to build support for local public health action, and develop local participatory approaches to health and environmental issues. The advocacy may well include major health and environment campaigns on the most urgent public health issues of the day, for example, cholera prevention where both the environmental as well as the personal health aspects would need to be addressed in a co-ordinated and integrated way. However a virtue of the healthy city approach is that it allows many different health and environment issues to be addressed through an ongoing process of developing and implementing a comprehensive city health plan.

INTRODUCING THE WHO'S HEALTHY CITY PROGRAMME

Definition of a Healthy City

'A Healthy City is one that is continually creating and improving those physical and social environments and expanding those community resources which enable people to mutually support each other in performing all the functions of life and in developing to their maximum potential' (Goldstein and Kickbusch 1996: p4).

Box 1.4 Core Healthy City Concepts

- Better health will come, not so much from curative care but from improved living conditions
- People must take the initiative to improve their own health and their own environments
- Health should be seen as an essential part of overall development within the community

Source: Goldstein and Kickbusch (1996)

The Healthy City Project is experiencing considerable popularity around the world, with at least 1,000 cities or towns adopting the Project. There are networks of healthy cities in all regions of the world, with anglophone, francophone, Spanish-speaking and Arabic-speaking networks linking different continents. The approach is based on the principle that health can be improved by modification of living conditions: the physical environment, and the social and economic conditions of everyday life. This holistic view sees health as the outcome of all the factors and activities which impinge upon the lives of individuals and communities.

Many city leaders, professionals and citizens have taken up the challenge to link up with a network of healthy cities in every region of the world, and to open up and develop the dimension of city level work in international public health. On the basis of experience in some 1,000 cities, Healthy City was presented to the Habitat II Human Settlements Summit in 1996 as an example of best practice in urban management.

The WHO, from its beginning in 1948, has recognized the interaction of physical, mental and social factors in determining health. In 1978, the WHO launched a major public health movement called 'Health for All' at Alma Ata, based on six principles (see Box 1.1). The Healthy City Project builds on the WHO's definition of health, and it has roots in the public health culture of many parts of the world, such as the local health systems in Latin America, the 'Health-Culture' movement in Japan, and, as already noted, the Ottawa Charter for Health Promotion.

In 1986, the European office of the WHO proposed a health promotion project to be known as the Healthy City Project. The intention of the Project was to devise ways to apply the principles and strategies of Health for All through local action in cities and put it on the agenda of local government.

In healthy city work attention is given to 'health opportunities'. Though various urban development activities (housing, industry, infrastructure, etc) can bring health hazards if they lack health and environmental safeguards, more importantly they offer health opportunities. They can enhance the health status of the population if health promotion and protection measures are undertaken in implementing the development. For example, in industrial development, safety considerations in factories and workshops, worker training and pollution control should be integral; or in housing development, water and sanitation and garbage services, and basic health care measures should be implemented with community participation.

A healthy city project supports city health authorities and/or local government in undertaking what may be two new roles:

- information and analysis – health impacts are monitored, involving measurement of health status and estimation of the contribution that various environmental factors are making to health problems. This is then followed by analysis of health requirements and opportunities in various development sectors that are significant for health;
- policy and advocacy – specific health policies for each sector are formulated (for water, sanitation, local government, education, industry, labour (for example, workplace health, etc), and are advocated by policy makers in the work of competent agencies.

In order to respond to the current interest in the healthy city movement in developing countries the remainder of this book's structure follows the various phases involved in healthy city projects, namely start-up, organization, implementation, data-gathering/priority setting and evaluation. A separate chapter is dedicated to sustainability of healthy city projects as this has emerged as a key issue. A concluding chapter then considers the future of healthy cities in developing countries.

2 Establishing Healthy City Projects

As noted in the introductory chapter, the Healthy City Project is an integrated, city-wide initiative. The process of establishing a healthy city project is delicate and elaborate, as it involves changes in institutional organization and enhancing intersectoral action. The latter often means that co-operative activities are undertaken by a number of key players, particularly local authorities, NGOs, citizen groups, and the national and provincial agencies that operate locally. Such issues may be problematic, especially when they challenge well entrenched behaviour and conditions, which is often the case in developing countries. The aim of this chapter is to analyse the constraints encountered in the process of establishing healthy city projects, and to discuss solutions to them.

The WHO has developed a set of guidelines to orient the setting up of healthy city projects (see for instance WHO 1995a). The cities and towns which have joined the healthy city movement lately, especially the ones in developing countries, have tended to follow them. Therefore, this chapter begins with the presentation of these guidelines as background information. It follows with a discussion of the main constraints for the implementation of the Project, and presents evidence from Chittagong and Quetta. The Chittagong Project was initiated in 1993, and is one of the first healthy city projects in the developing world. Since then, a number of evaluation exercises have been carried out to monitor progress. Such exercises have been valuable not only to correct on-going problems in Chittagong, but also as background information for healthy city projects elsewhere. The Quetta Project was initiated in 1995 and the analysis here shows how some of the constraints encountered in Chittagong were avoided in Quetta. The chapter also discusses further constraints that still need to be addressed, and their possible resolutions.

BASIC ELEMENTS OF THE PROCESS

WHO guidelines indicate that the institutional organization of a healthy city project should be based on a steering committee, a project office and working groups (WHO 1995a). The implementation of the project should follow three basic stages and be guided by the City Health Plan (sometimes called the Municipal Health Plan or the Healthy City Plan of Action) (CCC–WHO 1993; WHO 1995b). The health sector has an important, but not overwhelming, role in such a process. These issues will be elaborated on next.

The Institutional Organization of a Healthy City Project

The Steering Committee

A healthy city requires intersectoral action. It is therefore necessary to establish an interdisciplinary steering committee (sometimes also called a co-ordination council) to guide it. This committee is formed by members of various organizations which are involved in different aspects of the development of the city (see Box 2.1, for an illustration from Chittagong). It is generally presided over by the leading authority of the local government (ie the mayor or chairman). It is the supreme authority within each healthy city, and has the final say on any policy or action. Its roles include the approval of the City Health Plan; the decisions about any future amendment proposed by working groups to be included in the City Health Plan; actions on all emerging problems; actions to raise resources for implementing the Plan; to challenge constantly the working groups to widen their membership in order to strengthen partnerships between the government departments, the community and the NGOs.

Box 2.1 The Steering Committee of the Chittagong Healthy City Project

President:
- The Honourable Mayor, Chittagong City Corporation

Member Secretary:
- Chief Executive Officer, Chittagong City Corporation

Members:
- Chairmen, Chittagong Port Authority, Chittagong Water and Sewerage Authority and Chittagong Development Authority
- General Manager, Bangladesh Railway, Chittagong
- Police Commissioner, Chittagong Metropolitan Police
- Deputy Commissioner, Chittagong
- Principal, Chittagong Medical College
- Chairman, Department of Sociology, University of Chittagong
- Chief Engineer, Power Development Board, Chittagong
- Director, Directorate General of Health Services, Chittagong
- Conservator of Forests, Chittagong
- President, Chamber of Commerce and Industry, Chittagong
- General Managers, Bakharabad Gas System Ltd – Chittagong, and Telegraph and Telecommunications – Chittagong
- Superintending Engineer, Department of Public Health Engineering, Chittagong Circle
- Civil Surgeon, Chittagong
- Director, Department of Environment, Chittagong
- Deputy Directors, Education Directorates, Chittagong
- Project Director, Youth Development Directorate, Chittagong
- Project Director, Housing and Settlement Directorate, Chittagong
- Regional Director, Radio Bangladesh, Chittagong
- General Manager, Export Processing Zone, Chittagong
- Deputy Director, Women Affairs Directorate, Chittagong
- President, Press Club, Chittagong
- Representatives from WHO, UNICEF and UNDP
- Regional Officer, ADAB, Chittagong
- Area Manager, World Vision of Bangladesh, Chittagong
- Regional Officer, NGO Forum for Drinking Water Supply and Sanitation
- President, Lions Club and Rotary Club, Chittagong
- Ward Commisioners

Source: CCC–WHO (1993)

The Project Office

This office supports the steering committee, and is the operational arm of a healthy city project. It has a co-ordinator at its centre, generally with supporting staff and finances. The project office needs a physical basis (ie a room or set of rooms) with the necessary equipment for:

- the daily activities of the co-ordinator and his/her staff;
- the periodical meetings of the steering committee, the working groups and any other meeting necessary for the development of a healthy city project; and
- the collection of all relevant information about the project, which should be available for public consultation.

The roles of the project office include:

- awareness raising and community consultation to ensure that the views of citizens are fully taken into account in project development and implementation;
- ensuring that priorities and deadlines set by the steering committee are met;
- ensuring that the steering committee members are adequately supported;
- ensuring the overall development of the project, with constant encouragement of all the partners involved;
- developing a local action programme of specific demonstration projects (which involve partnerships between the local organizations and residents);
- developing capacity-building schemes (ie appropriate training courses for relevant people);
- arranging seminars and conferences;
- co-ordinating publicity for the project;
- networking with other healthy city projects;
- monitoring and assessing activities;
- developing sources of information on health issues.

The project co-ordinator plays the key role within the office. There have been successful co-ordinators from different backgrounds and different work experiences. For instance, the first co-ordinator in Chittagong was a magistrate. The second and present co-ordinator there is an engineer while the first co-ordinator in Quetta was a medical doctor.

Working Groups

The most common type of working group is constituted by the sectoral task forces, which are responsible for the specific plans and actions related to the different sectors of activity in the city *and their connection to the health of the population*. Some projects have also included zonal task forces, which are responsible for the specific plans and actions in each geographical area of the city. However, the use of sectoral task forces has prevailed.

There are endless ways of dividing and labelling the sectoral task forces. The partners of each healthy city project decide which is the best way to do it in their specific city or town. However, regardless of how the grouping will be made and which labels will be given, ideally all aspects of urban development should be included in the sectoral task forces. This is the case in the two cities studied in this chapter. Chittagong divided its task forces into seven:

(1) Town Planning, Infrastructure and Economic Development;
(2) Primary Health Care and Maternal and Child Health;
(3) Literacy and Unemployment;
(4) Water and Sewerage;
(5) Drainage and Sanitation;
(6) Environmental Protection; and
(7) Slum Improvement.

Quetta started with one overall task force, which constituted the embryo of the several task forces to be formed later on. Now there are seven task forces, organized in a different way than Chittagong's:

(1) Environmental Health Services;
(2) Housing and Land Development;

(3) Roads, Transport and Energy;
(4) Economic Development;
(5) Education;
(6) Social Affairs; and
(7) Health Services.

It is important to note that the sectoral task forces are not counterparts of municipal public departments, which operate solely within the structure of the local government. A given task force, by definition, includes representatives of all sectors of society which are somehow involved with a given field of activity. Therefore, it includes representatives of all the public agencies involved in such a field, plus representatives of the private sector (for example, chambers of commerce and industry), NGOs, community organizations, international agencies operating in town and academic institutions (WHO 1995a).

Healthy city projects also include actions which involve more than one task force. In such cases, each task force will be responsible for a component of the overall action, and should liaise with the other task forces involved in the same action.

Rather than focusing on all sectors of urban development and health, some cities have opted to concentrate on selected settings of everyday life (for example, house and neighbourhood, schools, workplaces, food markets) or specific issues such as accidents, crime and violence, pollution, or major disease problems. Examples include Accra, Ghana (which has focused on healthy schools) and Mandalay, Myanmar (focusing on children's health), among others. Other places, such as Campinas, Brazil, have chosen a zonal task force structure, but opted to concentrate in only one area of the city. It is fundamental for a healthy city project to have a systemic vision of urban development and health, as well as an integrated approach, even if it opts for very specific actions, such as in Accra, Mandalay and Campinas. This vision and approach will distinguish such healthy city actions from the myriad of specific projects that are routinely implemented in a fragmented way.

The Phases of a Healthy City Project

WHO guidelines have recommended that a healthy city project should be divided into three phases: start-up, organization and implementation. The start-up phase aims to initiate the process, to build wide public support for the project and to start awareness raising campaigns. During this phase the co-ordinator should be appointed. The major groups and organizations in the city that may take part in the project are contacted and encouraged to participate. During the second phase, the institutional organization of the project and the approval of the government authorities are consolidated. Also, the City Health Plan is produced. The third phase is devoted to the implementation of the City Health Plan, evaluation and setting-up of networks with other healthy city projects (WHO 1995a).

The City Health Plan

This Plan is of vital importance, as its design and implementation constitute the crux of the operations of a healthy city project. The project office has responsibility for the development of the Plan, which requires inputs from all the actors in the project. There are two basic types of input:

(1) the views of involved communities on their needs and priorities, so that the local perceptions of problems and issues are fully expressed; and
(2) a technical assessment based on available health statistics and known epidemiological linkage of the health status to the environmental and social conditions. Both of these assessments must be combined in the course of the development of the City Health Plan.

The Plan shows how the current living conditions in the city/town are affecting the health of the inhabitants, sets out principles for action, sets out the major challenges which the city/town will face to improve its health status, and proposes priorities and the ways in which they will be taken forward in a co-ordinated and systematic

Healthy City Projects in Developing Countries

way by the project partners (see Chapter 3). Ideally the Plan will cover each aspect of city development, and its relationship with the health of the population. The Plan should involve community participation in all aspects (from evaluation of needs to the implementation of action), and should be flexible enough to accommodate periodic amendments to respond to unexpected events. Box 2.2 includes a general outline for a City Health Plan. Table 2.1 includes a 'snapshot' of the Chittagong Health Plan (ie parts of the plan of action of one of the task forces).

Box 2.2 Outline of a Municipal Health Plan

This is based on the development of municipal health plans (MHPs) in the cities of Rio de Janeirio, Accra and Lahore during 1991/2.

Who formulates the plan?
A multisectoral team of community representatives and organizations including Ministry of Health (MOH) staff, NGOs the university, a representative from the mayor's office and representatives of hospitals and the media. The plan is consistent with national urban health/planning guidelines of the MOH and of ministries of urban development, and is endorsed by the mayor.

Goals of the plan

- To get health education and the other health-related activities incorporated into the community-level activities of municipal staff working in water, sanitation, solid waste, housing, education, social support and other areas; and
- to improve the performance of the municipality both in provision of services and in supporting local community initiatives and greater community participation in activities that promote health.

Prerequisites

- Community organization and representation in formulation of the plan.

- Health leadership, which may be found in the MOH, NGO or municipal office.
- A public hearing to allow broad public discussion.

Content

- Identify and review all studies and reports that are available that describe and quantify the social, economic and environmental health problems and environmental conditions in the city;
- attempt to rank the contribution that problems make to the burden of ill health;
- identify the existing municipal agencies and organizations, including UN bilateral agencies and NGOs, that can potentially contribute to solutions to health problems; and
- identify and rank the priority actions and programmes, including setting of targets, and evaluation plans.

Ensure action

- Commitment of community leaders;
- training of municipal staff and community participants;
- publish stories and reports in local media;
- monitor, evaluate and publish annual health status and activity data.

The MHP may have programmes or projects for specific settings, such as schools, workplaces, the market place and health care settings.

In preparing the plan, the project staff must keep in mind that there may be some government functions (policy making, services) that are outside the responsibility of the city government and are controlled by national ministries. Identification of these functions will be critical, as will information about which city and national politicians and officials are sympathetic to health issues, or to the involvement of citizen groups in local government, and therefore may be prepared to support the project.

The MHP is collated and analysed by the project, and distributed in government agencies, NGOs and the public in one or more healthy city project meetings. The plan is not so much a blueprint but a tool to promote discussion and raise awareness that there are possibilities of changing living conditions in the city for the better, through co-operative efforts and partnerships.

Source: WHO (1995c: pp15–16)

Table 2.1 *A 'Snapshot' of the Chittagong Health Plan: Part of the Plan of Action of the Water and Sewerage Task Force*

Action required	Organizations involved	Timescale
Support and assist the interim water supply project. This will rehabilitate the water supply from 20 deep tubewells, resulting in an additional 40 mgd supply by 1995. NGOs and WASA (Water and Sanitation Development Authority) will work together on a community mobilization education programme.	Led by WASA support by NGO Forum/ADAB (Association of the Development Agencies of Bangladesh).	With effect from November 1993. Report activities to the meeting by December 1995.
Advocate for the strengthening of WASA particularly in the fields of system loss, administration, management and revenue collection.	Led by WASA.	With effect from November 1995. Report to the next meeting.
To take resolution permitting different NGOs and the DPHE to provide water in the fringe areas where such facilities do not exist.	Led by CCC (Chittagong City Corporation) /WASA/ DPHE (Department of Public Health Engineering)/ NGO Forum.	By end of 1995.
Initiate a joint pilot programme between CCC and WASA to commercialize water hydrants in the Lalkhan Bazar.	CCC/WASA.	January 1996.
Develop a pollution testing programme for the Kalurghat Industrial Estate, the effluent from which flows into Halda River which provides two thirds of the city's surface water supply.	DOE (Department of the Environment)/ WASA.	January 1996.
Initiate feasibility study on extension and expansion of existing Mohara treatment plant.	WASA.	January 1996.
Assist with the implementation of GOB (Government of Bangladesh) targets for sewerage in Chittagong.	WASA/CCC/CPA (Chittagong Port Authority)/ CDA (Chittagong Development Authority).	Preliminary statement on target May 1996.
Act as a mechanism for the implementation of UNICEF Plan of Action on Basic Services for Women and Children.	UNICEF to lead all partners.	With immediate effect.
Make a feasibility survey of a small bore sewerage system for selected parts of the city.	WASA.	October 1995.

Source: CCC–WHO (1993)

Creating a Vision

In the process of consultation with the community and many different agencies and groups, there is an effort made to develop a vision of the future direction of the city, and to understand its current (and past) strengths and qualities. A 'Vision Workshop' may be held for this purpose, that can start with the question: 'why is this city a fine place to live?' In all parts of the world an appreciation of the cultural heritage, and cultivation of a 'sense of place' that celebrates the unique characteristics and history of each city is providing an important element in mobilizing people to improve living conditions and address health and environment problems.

The Role of the Health Sector

Considering that the Healthy City Project is about 'health', one would expect the so-called health sector to assume a prominent role on it (ie vis-à-vis all the other sectors, such as housing, transport, environment, etc). This is reinforced by the fact that the WHO has traditionally worked closely with the Ministry of Health, which is the head agency of the health sector in a country. However, as already seen, the Healthy City Project is very much linked with local government, and places a strong emphasis on intersectoral action. Therefore, what is the role of the health sector?

Many countries around the world have been relatively slow to develop coherent health policies to address health conditions in urban areas. Reasons for this may be:

- policies are increasingly needed outside the health sector to deal with the new and expanded areas of energy, agriculture, industrialization and advanced technology;
- gaps in knowledge related to the complexity of urban ill health; and
- the perception that there is insufficient evidence on which to act (Editorial 1996).

The health sector in many ways has simply not been able to keep up with the development of policies for other sectors. It is perhaps understandable in this context why intersectoral co-ordination for health has not been more forthcoming. Why, for example, would the transport or housing sector wish to engage another sector (health) which all too often has not measured the health burden of transport or housing sector activities, and therefore has little to say to them? In principle, the health authority has a key role to help ensure that the policies and activities of various sectors and organizations contribute positively to health protection and promotion. This requires it to help develop health policies for various sectors outside health services.

The development of an overall health policy, and of basic uniform environmental health standards, is a critical function which may be best co-ordinated by a national health authority. But other sectors and tiers of government need to be involved. For example, the role of a department of the environment would be to ensure that the policies and standards developed for various environmental health aspects of pollution control are consistent with overall environmental policy. Of equal importance is that implementation strategies – and not only the agenda – are developed in partnership with relevant agencies (Walker 1994).

Around the world there are many examples of public and environmental health possibilities that have gradually been eroded from under the control of health authorities, for example, food safety, meat inspection, chemical safety, waste management and pollution control. This erosion is particularly frequent in countries where environmental ministries and departments have been set up. The public health sector has lost organizational responsibility for many health and environmental activities at the national, regional and local levels (Gordon 1992). One reason why some health authorities have acquiesced to this loss is because environmental health is perceived as something negative, causing endless problems which are unmanageable, the roots of which frequently lie outside the health sector's direct responsibility. What attention should health authorities be directing to environmental health, given their increasing pressures and responsibilities to deal with all manner of pressing health problems and diseases? Should the mandate of health authorities be expanded to address more fully the wide spectrum of health and environmental challenges, or should it be narrowed and more focused? Is the health sector in the business of environmental control, and if so in what way? (Gordon 1991). The Healthy City Project is a vehicle through which the health sector can respond to these challenges.

While an intersectoral policy for cities requires that public and environmental health should be part of the responsibility of all development sectors, the health sector (in particular the national health authority) has the following essential roles:

- Monitoring of overall (environmental) health status at city, neighbourhood and district levels, including ensuring that intra-urban and intra-district differences are detected (this is important in terms of shifting the focus of regulatory control in many countries from low risks which often affect only relatively small percentages of the population).
- Estimating the contribution that various environmental and social factors are making to health problems, using improved indicators of the relationship between health and living conditions to support decision makers.
- Analysing environmental and social health needs and requirements in various development sectors that are significant for health, such as housing, local government, transport, industry and so on, with consideration of the health opportunities offered by each sector.
- Formulating specific public health and environmental health policies, health-related legislation, standards and targets, in partnership with each sector (such as for water, sanitation, local government, education, industry, labour).
- Advocating, facilitating and enabling health issues to be addressed in the work of competent agencies, organizations and communities at all levels, and promoting health and environment generally.
- Supporting regional and local environmental health service delivery and providing such services that cannot feasibly be provided by other tiers of government.

- Supporting the development of research which may be necessary in order to better understand, assess and manage environmental health risks.
- Providing technical support and guidance in policy and planning, evaluation, and capacity development.

The above areas require intersectoral co-operation, as opposed to the more traditional functions of the health sector in the areas of diagnosis, treatment and rehabilitation. They depend fundamentally on the need for partnerships to promote intersectoral, intergovernmental, interdisciplinary and community action for health. Thus intersectoral co-operation is necessary in the areas of advocacy, health impact and risk assessment, epidemiological surveillance, policy and planning, among others.

ISSUES FOR DISCUSSION

The basic elements necessary for the implementation of a healthy city project, as suggested by the WHO, have been presented above. The use of general guidelines in different contexts, however, often requires adaptations. As already mentioned, the Healthy City Project entails changes in institutional behaviour, which may face constraints especially when they challenge well entrenched conditions. The analysis of healthy city projects in developing countries revealed the existence of such constraints, thus demonstrating the need for adaptations in the general guidelines. The analysis developed here concentrates on three sets of interrelated issues.

The first set regards the public sector. It focuses on whether the institutional organization of public authorities is appropriate for the implementation of a healthy city project, whether the local government has the necessary leadership for the political guidance of the project, and whether the relationships within the public sector are conducive to a successful implementation of the project. A discussion of these issues is important because a healthy city project must address the public sector and use the office of the local government in order to ensure city wide implementation. The aim here is to identify and analyse constraints for the participation of the public sector.

The second set of issues regards the insertion of the project in the city/town. This set focuses on whether the healthy city concept has been understood by the local stakeholders; how to pool resources for the implementation of the project; whether there is scope formally to merge the project with existing policies; and whether the project office has the capacity to co-ordinate all the actions.

Finally, the third set regards the non-public stakeholders, thus including partnerships with community and popular organizations, NGOs, the private sector and international agencies. This issue is important because wide participation of the different sectors of society and partnerships between different stakeholders is essential for healthy cities. All three sets of interrelated issues are elaborated next, with illustrations from Chittagong and Quetta.

CASE STUDIES

Chittagong is an ancient city, which remained small until 1960, when it had an area of 10.24 sq km and a population of 300,000. In the past few decades Chittagong has experienced rapid growth. In 1993 it had an area of 183.4 sq km, and the population was between 1.5 and 2.5 million. The city is now the second largest in Bangladesh, its main sea port and main industrial centre (CCC–WHO 1993). However, similar to most cities in the developing world, the growth of Chittagong has been accompanied by increasing urban problems. Poverty abounds, and it is estimated that there are 110 slum areas in the city, with some 1 million inhabitants (CCC–WHO 1993). The provision of most urban services has been deficient, and the built fabric shows many signs of decay.

Quetta, the capital city of the Province of Balochistan in Pakistan, takes its name from the ancient citadel called 'Kwatta' or 'Kota' in Pashto, which was built where the city now stands to protect the strategic crossing roads to Afghanistan, Persia (Iran) and India. Until late in the 19th century Quetta was still predominantly a military outpost. Under British rule Quetta grew in importance due to its strategic location. It kept its military function and gradually incorporated other roles, for example, market town, railhead, site of the imperial staff college in British India. The development of Quetta suffered a great setback in 1935 when an earthquake destroyed the town and killed around 20,000 people. After this disaster Quetta was rebuilt and resumed its growth. In 1981 its population was 286,167. Since that year the town has experienced a large growth mainly due to migration from Afghanistan and from the rural areas of Balochistan. Its current estimated population is around 1 million. The magnitude and the pattern of this growth has brought pressure on the provision of most urban services.

The Chittagong Healthy City Project started with a series of meetings and workshops in 1993, sponsored by the WHO. The Quetta Project started in 1995. A number of evaluations of these projects have been carried out in order to monitor progress (for example, Werna 1994, 1995a, 1995b, 1996a, 1996b). Such evaluations have produced findings which illustrate the issues highlighted in the beginning of the previous section.

The Institutional Organization of Public Authorities

Traditional structures of local government have been based on compartmental administration with few or no horizontal connections between different areas or services, and with a strong emphasis on the role of the public bureaucracy. However, in the past few decades there has been a move towards a flexible structure of urban management, with an emphasis on integration between areas or services as well as on the co-operation between the public sector and the other actors involved with urban management (for example, Devas and Rakodi 1993; Stoker 1990; Werna 1995c, 1995d). These trends are currently more advanced in industrialized countries. Although there has been some evidence of moves in this direction in developing countries, they are still incipient. Such trends are not advanced in Chittagong and Quetta (Werna 1994, 1995a, 1995b). For instance:

> 'The verticalised-bureaucratised structure encountered in the organisation of the urban government [of Chittagong] in general, as already noted, is replicated within the City Corporation. According to the analysis carried out by BKH (1989, 1990), there is no inter-departmental, inter-sector and inter-ward coordination; performance monitoring and reporting systems. There is also a wide variation of management structure for analogous kinds

of services. This was confirmed through the interviews carried out by the author. Another issue unveiled in the interviews is that the City Corporation officers have a weak tradition of team work' (Werna 1994: pp7–8).

However, as the WHO puts it, the Healthy City Project condemns the traditional systems of organization, rooted in 'concepts of bureaucracy, hierarchy, paternalistic power, professional authority, disciplinary specialisation, win–lose and either/or strategy and sectoral analysis' (WHO 1991: pp12–13). Therefore, '[T]o address the problems of the 21st century, however... new, holistic, flexible approaches [must be] adopted' (WHO 1991: pp12–13).

These new approaches

'cut across the old departmental lines and indeed across the different sectors – public, private, voluntary and community. None can be addressed by one department of government alone, nor indeed by city government alone. The whole community has to be mobilised and the efforts of all sectors and departments have to be combined and focused' (WHO 1991: pp12–13).

The WHO also notes that 'some of these changes have already been under way for 20 years or more' (WHO 1991: p13). However, this statement is based on the reality of industrialized countries. As already mentioned, the situation in developing countries is often not the same. The cases of Chittagong and Quetta have shown that the local authorities have not had the necessary structure to absorb fully the innovations brought by the Healthy City Project. This will be illustrated by a number of issues explained below. Under such circumstances, the Healthy City Project may have an important role as a vehicle for change. However, it is necessary to bear in mind that it will require a longer period for implementation.

Institutional Leadership of the Project

The local government has been regarded as the institution which should lead the Project in each city or town. The WHO suggests that the mayor should head the steering committee, top officials of the local government should have prominence in the several task forces and the project office should be located within the local government premises. It is important, however, to see if the local government has the necessary power to enforce its leadership. Although decentralization is now a key word in public administration throughout developing countries, real devolution of power to local government has seldom taken place. Chittagong and Quetta are no exceptions.

The Chittagong Healthy City Project is being implemented under the responsibility of the Chittagong City Corporation (ie the local government). However, there are more than 20 public agencies connected to eight different ministries involved in several aspects of the administration of the city and in the provision of its public services (see Box 2.3). These agencies are not under the command of the City Corporation and there is no alternative co-ordinating body. As a result, problems of lack of co-operation and co-ordination take place, such as overlap of functions in some areas and deficiencies in others.

Box 2.3 The Hand of Central Government in Chittagong

Selected public agencies accountable to the central government and responsible for the provision of urban services in Chittagong:

- Bakrabad Gas Company
- Bangladesh Institute of Technology
- Bangladesh Railway
- Bangladesh Road Transport Corporation
- Chittagong Development Authority
- Chittagong University
- Civil Surgeon
- Defence Service
- Department of Public Health Engineering
- Export Processing Zone
- Facilities Department
- Housing and Settlement Directorate
- Liquidified Petroleum Gas Plant
- Roads and Highway Department
- Port Authority
- Power Development Board
- Primary/Secondary/Higher Education Departments

> - Public Works Department
> - Technical Education Board
> - Water and Sewerage Authority
> - Water Development Board
>
> Source: Werna (1994)

In Quetta, the two primary local public agencies are the Quetta Municipal Corporation (QMC) and the Quetta Development Authority (QDA). Both agencies operate under the control of the Government of the Province of Balochistan. The QMC is the local government agency responsible for the overall management of the city, except the cantonment area and the peripheral areas which outstrip the municipal boundaries. At present it is run by an appointed administrator, not an elected mayor. The QDA is responsible for urban planning and development, and for building infrastructure (excluding the cantonment and the peripheral areas). The cantonment is managed separately under the control of the federal government. It comprises 14.7 per cent of Quetta's population. Public agencies from the provincial level of government (ie the Province of Balochistan) and from the district level (ie the District of Quetta, which encompasses the whole valley) also play a major role in the development of the city and its outskirts. The Planning and Development Department of Balochistan, for example, formulates economic and social policies for the whole province, co-ordinates the activities of all sectors, evaluates public investment projects and monitors allocations of the Annual Development Programme (ADP). The Local Government and Rural Development Department of Balochistan controls the local bodies, including the QMC. The Finance Department of Balochistan determines financial policies and controls loans, grants and budgetary support for all provincial agencies. This includes the provision of funds for the ADP activities of the QDA and occasional support for the QMC. District and provincial sectoral agencies (responsible for health services, education, transport, etc) also play an important role in Quetta.

Relationships within the Public Sector

The relationship between different layers of government affect the cities' development in many ways (for example, Davey 1992). This is especially true in places such as Chittagong and Quetta, where, as noted above, the level of decentralization is still low.

The first mayor of Chittagong to be directly elected by the city's population took power in early 1994. The previous mayors were appointed by the central government, and therefore there was a political alignment between central and local government. The new mayor, however, was in opposition to the Prime Minister who held power until 1996: a fact that strained central–local relations during the 1994–1996 period (at present central and local governments are aligned again). Considering the increasing democratization of developing countries, tension in central–local relations is likely to take place in, and affect, other healthy city projects. This may also recur in Chittagong in the future, after a change in the current local and/or central governments.

In Quetta, at present, municipal administration is directly appointed by the provincial government – therefore there are no major tensions in the local–provincial governments' relations. However, such tensions may recur in the future, if or when the local government resumes its independence from the provincial government.

Healthy city projects have concentrated on building partnerships between intra-urban stakeholders. A notable exception regards ministries of health: most projects try to engage this ministry, for often there is no health authority within a city government and it is the ministry of health – outside and operating independently from the city government – that has responsibility for health. However, there is a need to extend such partnerships to further central or regional authorities, therefore involving central/provincial government policy makers and decision makers who influence urban matters. This has been done in Quetta since the onset of its Healthy City Project, by comprehensively involving the provincial government.

The traditional systems of public administration, which are widespread in developing countries, entail a lack of horizontal linkages not only at the local government level, but also at the central and provincial levels. As already noted, more than 20 public agencies which operate in Chittagong are directly accountable to eight different central ministries. Therefore, lack of co-ordination/co-operation among such ministries affects the Chittagong Project. This reinforces the need for acting at the central government level on behalf of the healthy city project. In Quetta, the provincial government has recognised the existence of conflicts between the activities of the different agencies operating in the city and it has constituted a committee

Establishing Healthy City Projects

to co-ordinate such activities. This is an important step, and the Healthy City Project will benefit enormously if fine co-ordination is achieved.

Conceptual Understanding of the Project

Healthy city projects entail organizational changes which are extremely innovative in many localities. In Chittagong the innovations brought by the Project have challenged not only the traditional behaviour of most local stakeholders, but also their expectations vis-à-vis international programmes. At the onset of the Chittagong Project, many local stakeholders regarded it as international/WHO top-down assistance to the city, and developed expectations about large sums of external funding, and the like. Subsequently, the assimilation of healthy city concepts, such as a reliance on local resources and a bottom-up approach, by the local partners of the Project proved to be difficult.

Therefore, it is necessary to bear in mind that the conceptual understanding of healthy cities is likely to encounter difficulties. The Quetta Project learned from the Chittagong experience, and addressed the issue from the beginning. While it is important to use the local media more often, it is also vital to use alternative methods of communication to reach the considerable portion of the population which does not have access to the formal media. UNICEF (present both in Chittagong and Quetta) and many NGOs have considerable experience in campaigns of dissemination which target these populations. They should be approached to help the Healthy City Project to design non-formal communication methods, in Chittagong, Quetta and elsewhere.

Resources

Among the peculiarities of developing countries, the issue of resources for the implementation of the City Health Plan is particularly worth noting. Healthy city projects in industrialized countries have a strong emphasis on pooling local resources to address each city or town's health issues – therefore assuming that each city/town somehow has the necessary resources to address its problems. In this respect, the task of a healthy city project is to find such resources and/or to organize them in an adequate way.

The idea of pooling local resources is of course applicable to developing countries, and indeed is a characteristic of healthy city projects in such parts of the world as well. However, the balance between problems and resources in the cities and towns in the developing world is considerably different from that of their counterparts in industrialized countries. By and large, while the latter have more resources to address fewer problems, the situation in the former is exactly the opposite. For instance, while healthy city projects such as Liverpool's or Glasgow's may be struggling to fill in gaps in their urban development plans; Chittagong and Quetta did not even have such a plan until recently. Healthy city projects in the North may be addressing pockets of poverty which still exist in their (at least relatively) wealthy urban areas. However, many cities in the South actually have a vast poor urban sprawl with pockets of wealth. In sum, cities/towns in developing countries often lack resources locally to address their problems comprehensively. Therefore, they often need external support.

However, the search for external support should by no means counteract the policy of pooling local resources, which is a basic premise of healthy city projects. As already noted, the Chittagong Project was affected by the local partners' over-reliance on external resources. Such a behaviour may lead at best to the adoption of a passive attitude in relation to the city's development, which is exactly the opposite of what Healthy City preaches. At worst it will lead to a stagnation in the city's development, considering the small size of the international bag of money vis-à-vis the demand of developing countries.

In sum, external resources should be obtained in a systematic manner. Such an issue has been highlighted in a number of WHO missions for healthy city projects in developing countries (this also includes an early mission to Quetta, to address the issue from the onset) (see for example, Werna, 1995e, 1996b). The idea is to encourage local partners first to use the local resources as thoroughly as possible, and only after such a stage should external resources be sought – first elsewhere in the country, and finally internationally. International resources should be sought only to meet needs that have been chosen as priorities for the healthy city project (the issue of priority selection will be approached in the next chapter). The local partners are also briefed about the likelihood of international donors appreciating applications for support which clearly demonstrate that local resources have already been thoroughly used, and that the items included in the application have been chosen as priorities via a city-wide consultation process. Considering the prominence of this issue for the implementation of healthy city projects in developing countries, it should be continuously emphasized.

Local Policies

The WHO states that the Healthy City Project seeks to build a strong case for public health at the local level, and to put health issues onto the agenda of urban policy makers. This statement implies that the Project has been implemented in cities and towns where the existing policies are deficient in addressing health issues as part of urban management and planning. Ideally, the Project should influence local policies to the point of being totally absorbed by them. At such a point, the Healthy City project would cease to exist as a specific project in the city/town, therefore becoming a permanent part of the local policy agenda.

In Chittagong, the type and degree of commitment of many local institutions to the Healthy City project has not been clear. This has led many local officials to perceive their activities related to the Project as voluntary or philanthropic, a fact which has undermined their commitment and efficiency. This is related to two issues already analysed; difficulty to accommodate the Project within a traditional organizational structure, and a difficulty in understanding its concepts. The germs of this problem have also been detected in Quetta. However, again Quetta benefited from the experience of Chittagong, and the issue has been addressed since the onset of the Quetta Project.

One should indeed expect conflicts between the Project activities and the day-to-day routines of the city's management, exactly because the Project challenges/innovates such routines. It is fundamental, however, to address such conflicts, or else the impact – and eventual blending – of the Project in the local policies will be jeopardized. Considering that the people who work in the local institutions are the very members of the Project (ie the steering committee, project office and the task forces), it is fundamental to harmonize thoroughly all their activities. It is important that the officials from the local institutions do not perceive the Healthy City Project as an extra burden. This entails raising their awareness, and linking the Project's activities as much as possible – and as early as possible – to the official activities of the various local institutions.

The Project Office

The project office has a strategic importance for a healthy city project, being its operational arm. It co-ordinates the plans and actions of all the project's partners. Ideally, the role of the office should be strictly managerial, considering that the partners are the people who implement the City Health Plan, through the task forces. However, if the partners/task forces face constraints, the co-ordinator of the project office has to play a more action-oriented role. As already noted, evidence from Chittagong has revealed the existence of constraints such as lack of understanding of the Project, lack of motivation and resources. Once these problems were detected, the co-ordinator in Chittagong was briefed to take such an action-oriented role. A similar briefing was made in Quetta, as a preventive measure.

The idea is that the co-ordinator should personally visit the different members/partners of the project to:

- motivate them;
- discuss the development of their on-going activities;
- co-ordinate such activities with those of the other partners;
- participate in solving any problems which might arise;
- plan future activities; and
- co-ordinate the planned and on-going actions of the other partners.

One possible way to do this would be via the establishment of a schedule of visits per sector of the healthy city project. The co-ordinator may start with one given task force. Thus, s/he should set aside a number of days to cover all its partners. The co-ordinator should keep a separate file for each partner, in which s/he will note the outcome of each visit (such a file is fundamental to review progress when the co-ordinator visits the partner again, later on). After completing the round of visits of the first task force, the co-ordinator should follow a similar procedure regarding the other forces. After completing all visits, the co-ordinator should start again, therefore generating a continuous process. In the second (and following) round(s) of visits the co-ordinator will be able to monitor progress, and to act accordingly. These rounds of visits obviously do not preclude the need for having occasional meetings with a whole task force, joint meetings with task forces and/or the steering committee.

The involvement of local governments of industrialized countries in healthy city projects has included, among other things, the setting up of the project office, ie contributing with physical facilities, furniture, equipment, and, especially, the cadre. There is indeed a rationale for such support. The project will only be sustainable if it is fully absorbed by the local partners, with the local government the main partner, as already noted. Also, the WHO is limited in its ability to pump funds into specific projects, especially considering the rising number of cities and towns joining the healthy city movement.

However, as the case of Chittagong demonstrates, a poorer city faces difficulties in supporting the project office. The initial office co-ordinator was financed by the City Corporation, but he could dedicate only a portion of his time to the Project's activities. He was also a public magistrate, which is a highly demanding occupation, and had to divide his time between this job and the co-ordination of the Project – the City Corporation claimed not to have funds to hire someone on a full time basis for the office. Therefore, the co-ordinator was constrained by shortage of time, a problem which was exacerbated by his lack of experience with healthy city projects.

The initial co-ordinator was replaced in 1995 by the executive engineer of the City Corporation. This second co-ordinator has shown a deeper understanding and commitment regarding the Project. However, the constraint of time persists, as he has also kept his previous job – and again the position of executive engineer is highly demanding. The reason the City Corporation maintains such a solution to the project office is the same as before, ie professed lack of funds to hire a full time co-ordinator.

Such a problem may be avoided in forthcoming healthy city projects if the local governments clearly understand, from the onset, the vital role of the project office, and the overwhelming difficulties that their projects will face without a full time, fully supported co-ordinator. Alternatively, other resources, if available, may be poured into the city to support the office and its co-ordinator until the project starts producing concrete results – assuming that at such a point the local authorities would be convinced about the importance of the healthy city project, and therefore of the advantages in supporting it. This latter suggestion is being applied in Quetta, as the WHO has managed to secure funds to sponsor a full time co-ordinator for three years.

It is also worth noting that the more the project blends into the local policies and routine actions, the less likely it is to remain an extra burden on the public resources. This should provide encouragement for making greater expenditures at the onset. But even if the local authorities fully realize the importance of the healthy city project, the problem would of course remain for the critical cases of extreme shortage of funds. In this respect, efforts should be made to try to find a local (co)sponsor for the project (thus reinforcing the importance of partnerships) rather than dropping the idea of having a full time co-ordinator.

Partnerships

Partnerships constitute a crux of healthy city projects. They may take place in different ways. For example, the project members realize that a given on-going activity is important to the City Health Plan, but the specific organization responsible for this activity may be experiencing difficulties in implementing it. Therefore, other project partners could offer their support to secure its full implementation. Another example regards the case of a number of partners who could pool resources to implement a future activity included in the City Health Plan. Alternatively, such partners could submit a joint proposal for external funding, in case local resources are not available. Other examples abound.

It is important to analyse the main partners of the Project. As the public sector has already been discussed, attention will now be given to community/popular organizations, NGOs, the private sector and international agencies.

Community/Popular Organizations
Community participation is a major foundation of the Healthy City Project (see, for example, Draper et al 1993; Petersen 1996). Current wisdom highlights its crucial importance in all aspects of urban development. However, the use of this concept has often encountered difficulties, which deserve examination.

The concept of community has often been associated with a geographical fix, for example, the community of a given shanty town, a village, a housing estate (see, for instance, Petersen 1996). Subsequently, community-based organizations (such as neighbourhood and shanty town associations) have often been regarded as the vehicle par excellence for community participation.

Also, the concept of community has frequently been associated with social cohesion and a readiness to participate. However, a number of recent studies about communities and their organizations have revealed a very different scenario, which includes exploitation of a (sub)group by another, lack of willingness to participate in matters related to the development of their locality, among other issues (see Petersen 1996, for a review). There is also specific evidence of such problems within healthy city projects in industrialized countries, associated with further problems such as top-down resistance against community participation, lack of information and other resources to enable a greater level of participation (for example, Petersen 1996; Tsouros 1990).

The above scenario is even more complicated in developing countries in many respects. For instance, high levels of illiteracy and scant resources for awareness raising and information campaigns make it difficult for communities to understand fully the concepts and routines of the healthy city project. There is often a lack of tradition of community participation, as well as resistance to it, especially (but not only) in authoritarian regimes. In this respect, one should note that Chittagong gained its first elected mayor only a few years ago, and Quetta does not have one at present.

The above reasoning may explain the recurring low level of community participation in Chittagong, and also suggests that it is likely to take place in Quetta (it is still too early to evaluate participation in this city). While community participation may be highly desirable in healthy city projects, it is fundamental to understand its associated problems, and to act accordingly.

It is also worth noting the difference between community participation and popular participation – two concepts which are often used synonymously. The former is often associated with a geographical fix, as already noted. The latter, in its turn, entails wider participation by different means/channels, which may include, but are not restricted to, community participation. The (broader) concept of popular participation may not be devoid of problems. However, it includes more options through which participation may be realized, leading to greater flexibility to adapt to local circumstances. An interesting idea that has been discussed in the Quetta Project is the formation of a Citizen's Forum, which would have a representative in the Project's steering committee. A counterpart in Chittagong is the Slum Dwellers' Forum (which constitutes a poor people's forum). Both are still incipient, and deserve full support to address the problems examined above. Special attention should be given to methods of dealing with citizens, groups, communities and leaders who do not have experience of participatory exercises. On the other hand, if the 'initial friction' is overcome, the Project itself may become a good vehicle and forum for the establishment of a participatory praxis.

NGOs

NGOs have gained wide prominence in urban development assistance, as they cater for an important share of the basic demands of the poor. This has been confirmed by evidence from healthy city projects in developing countries – there are some 30 NGOs operating in Chittagong, and 20 in Quetta (Werna 1994, 1995a, 1995b). Also, the role of NGOs in healthy city projects is likely to increase further, due to the current liaison between this Project and the Local Initiative for the Environment (LIFE) Programme of the United Nations Development Programme (UNDP) (the LIFE Programme gives funds for NGOs to develop urban environment-related activities).

In the beginning, the Chittagong Project encountered some resistance from a number of NGOs, which were concerned about the ownership of their specific activities (Werna 1994). This issue deserves attention. The Healthy City Project also includes the integration of individual activities, and the support for such activities to contribute as much as possible to the development of the city/town and the improvement of the health situation of its population. Considering that such individual activities are implemented by particular organizations (NGOs, public agencies, private firms, etc), one may wonder whether they would lose their rights, ownership and the credit over their individual activities, in favour of the Healthy City Project. This should not take place.

For example, suppose that a given NGO has implemented a housing scheme in one slum area. The Healthy City Project would stimulate this NGO to use the scheme as much as possible to address health problems related to its specific field (housing, in the case of this example), and would make an effort to link such an activity to other on-going and planned activities of the City Health Plan. However, this does not mean that the authorship and the rights of the housing scheme will be 'taken away' from the NGO.

The above clarification was later re-emphasized to the NGOs in Chittagong. Also, precautions in this respect have been taken in the Quetta Project since its onset, to avoid misunderstandings that could jeopardize partnerships.

The existence of umbrella organizations within the NGO sector in Chittagong and Quetta have helped to co-ordinate the liaison between this sector and the Healthy City Project – these organizations include the Association of Development Agencies of Bangladesh and the Balochistan NGOs Federation, respectively. Such umbrella organizations should be approached, or their constitution encouraged, in other healthy city projects.

At present NGOs have a prominent reputation in the development assistance scene. A number of international agencies and initiatives, in addition to the previously mentioned LIFE programme, are particularly interested in funding NGOs in developing countries. Therefore, the project offices, with the support of the WHO, could act as a liaison between potential donors and potential candidates.

The Private Sector

The private sector, in its turn, produces a significant share – and often the greater part – of the urban services and goods (especially considering that informal businesses are also part of the private sector). Considering the current widespread privatization policies and related trends throughout the world, the role of the private sector in urban development is due to remain significant, and even to increase. Such a role should not be underestimated in healthy city projects. However, evidence from Chittagong and Quetta shows that the participation of the private sector is still incipient. So far it has been limited to embryonic actions from organizations such as the Chamber of Commerce, Lions Club and Rotary Club. Recent suggestions to improve the situation include the setting up of deals in which a private enterprise would fund a given activity of the project (or part of it) in exchange for free publicity. Other possibilities should also be explored.

International Agencies

A large number of cities and towns in developing countries are hosts to international projects other than healthy city projects. Chittagong and Quetta are no exceptions. There are both multilateral and bilateral agencies operating in these cities, in parallel to the WHO. Co-ordination of such international projects is important, especially taking into consideration that local authorities in developing countries tend not to impose restrictions on international donors. Although such an attitude may be understandable where there is a shortage of local resources, it should not drive the

> authorities to the other extreme, as the concomitant implementation of different projects without thorough planning may lead to conflicts and wastage of resources.
>
> Considering the holistic character of the healthy city project, it has great scope for integrating the actions of the international agencies between themselves as well as with the local stakeholders' actions. In this context, advocacy for the involvement of the international agencies may be made both in town, by the healthy city partners, and in the international arena, by the WHO.

CONCLUSION

This chapter has shown that the Chittagong and Quetta Projects have been established under conditions which are in many respects different from those of industrialized countries. Therefore, it notes the importance of adapting the healthy city project to developing countries. It also notes that the evaluation of the Chittagong Project has been valuable not only to correct on-going problems in this city, but also to avoid them in Quetta. Furthermore, the chapter has discussed constraints that still need to be addressed in both cities. A set of actions to address such constraints has been recommended.

The Healthy City Project is an international (ie WHO) project, a fact which entails external inputs to the cities/towns, including the Project's design and start-up, among others. At the same time, Healthy City projects have a strong bottom-up/local reliance ethos. Therefore, the WHO and other international partners need to keep a balance between spoon-feeding the cities/towns, and starving them of inputs.

The overall analysis developed in this chapter may be useful as an initial check-list for detecting and avoiding constraints in forthcoming projects. Considering that other international initiatives bear a number of similarities with healthy city projects – especially the ones which also have an integrated/holistic approach – a number of issues here analysed may be pertinent to them as well, for instance, constraints such as concept understanding, resistance of traditional organizations, partnerships, inadequacy of local policies and resources. Currently there is a strong emphasis on integrated/holistic programmes of urban development in multilateral agencies (see, for example, Werna 1996c). However, considering that concrete experiences of implementation are still scant, findings from healthy cities will be of great value.

Considering that the establishment of the Healthy City Project in the developing world is still incipient, it would be interesting to set up a programme of comparative evaluation of experiences in this set of countries (Chapter 4 includes suggestions on how to carry out a comparative evaluation exercise). This would place each project in a broader context and at the same time would counteract the present tendency of making references to industrialized countries. In the long run, such a comparative work would systematically unveil the similarities and differences between healthy city projects in developing countries – thus identifying the issues which may or may not be emulated or generalized.

The present chapter highlighted that, among the peculiarities of developing countries, the issue of resources for the implementation of the City Health Plan is particularly worth noting. The balance between problems and resources in the cities/towns in the developing world is notably different from that of their counterparts in industrialized countries. Generally, while the latter have more resources to address fewer problems, the situation in the former is precisely the opposite. Therefore, in a situation of scarce resources, it is fundamental to devise thorough ways of establishing priorities for action. This is a fundamental issue in the process of implementation of healthy city projects, which will be analysed in the following chapter.

3 Implementing Healthy City Projects

INTRODUCTION

The previous chapter outlined some of the processes involved in establishing a healthy city project. It considered various issues pertinent to the start-up and organization phases. This chapter will consider the implementation of healthy city projects. It will look into how the City Health Plans mentioned in Chapter 2 are devised and further developed and it will explore the types of actions that might be involved in a healthy city project. In addition, the chapter will provide examples of the implementation of healthy city projects in three locations: Fayoum in Egypt, Quetta in Pakistan and Campinas in Brazil.

Implementing a healthy city project involves the creation and adoption of a City Health Plan. This involves four related processes:

- linking health status to environmental conditions;
- information gathering;
- priority setting; and
- action.

Although these processes are discussed separately, there are clear and important connections between them that will be demonstrated.

LINKING HEALTH STATUS TO ENVIRONMENTAL CONDITIONS

Linking health status to environmental conditions is fundamental to healthy city projects. It is an essential part of the process by which health policy moves away from a narrow consideration of what happens within the health services towards a broader consideration of how the activities of other sectors may have an effect on a population's health. It is now generally acknowledged that the environment (both physical, social and economic) exerts strong direct and indirect influences on health. Using this broad definition most of the problems faced by city dwellers can be classed as environmental. Problems related to the physical environment might include air and water pollution, excessive noise and overcrowded housing. Social environmental problems include lack of social support, the difficulty recent migrants from rural areas face in adapting to the urban setting, clashes between contrasting cultural and religious groups sharing densely populated districts and inequality between urban population groups. Economic problems relate to factors such as unemployment, job insecurity, low income, and lack of access to food and shelter. In some cases the mechanisms linking the environment and health are well documented: this usually occurs in the case of the relatively direct impacts involved in physical environment–health relationships, for example, polluted water and diarrhoeal diseases. In other cases the mechanisms are less clearly defined: this tends to occur in the case of indirect impacts involved in social environment–health relationships, for example, lack of good social support and common mental disorders. Dividing environmental factors into physical, social and economic factors is artificial and it is important to remember that the three are entwined: economic factors (for example income) often directly affect an individual or family's ability to prevent exposure to physical hazards.

Linking the effects of the physical, social and economic environment, Wilkinson (1996) draws on recent multi-disciplinary research and has shown how the effects of poverty are mediated through low social cohesion, marginalization of poor people and lack of social participation. The possibility has emerged that the serious health problems of poor people are not only the result of a lack of clean water, a decent house, sanitation and basic services. They also result from despair, anger, fear, worry about debts, worry about job and housing insecurity, feelings of failure and social alienation. He shows for example that the decline in social cohesion in Eastern Europe in the 1970s and 1980s is clearly related to the widening East–West mortality gap. The conclusion is that chronic stress – arising from social exclusion and devaluation as a human being – may be as damaging to health as the dangerous housing and working conditions poor people experience. Polarization, increased inequality and profound poverty not only violate basic principles of justice and fairness, they also breed alienation, despair and crime. More egalitarian societies connect people through a variety of social organizations, purposes and activities.

Environmental health impacts should be analysed in a broad development context, emphasizing the fact that it is important to develop indicators not only of health effects and their various causal or contributing risk factors at different levels, but also indicators for the assessment of various actions which might be taken to mitigate such problems. The linkage of health and environmental factors relies on methods for analysing grouped data, and many statistical methods are available, including ecological analysis, times series analysis and health risk analysis. Ecological analysis has been widely used in linkage work as it is relatively easy to undertake. For reasons of logistics and cost in many situations it may also be the only feasible approach. Until recently, times series analysis was not often applied in environmental epidemiology and linkage work, but it has now been recognized as a particularly useful element in linkage work. Health risk analysis requires data on exposures, together with estimates of the populations exposed, and of the health effects in the form of a dose-response function. These requirements have limited the applicability of health risk analysis. More recently geographical information systems (GIS) have become increasingly used as tools for manipulating spatial data and therefore of use in linkage analysis. GIS permits the controlled manipulation of data presented graphically, thereby revealing spatial patterns, irregularities or connections.

Often the capabilities of the local healthy city project staff or partners will determine the approaches and depth of the linkage analysis that is performed. A number of healthy city projects (for example Managua and Dar es Salaam) have adopted the HEADLAMP methodology to assist linkage and decision-support. HEADLAMP refers to the programme 'Health and Environment Analysis for Decision-making – Linkage Analysis and Monitoring Project' which involves the application of known exposure–disease relationships to new empirical data, as a basis for improved decision making and policy support. Corvalan et al (1997) and Briggs et al (1995) provide details of the conceptual and methodological issues in the approach, and in linkage work in general.

INFORMATION GATHERING

The WHO guidelines for healthy city projects include consideration of the information required for decision making. Indeed it is stated that 'It is essential to have a good understanding of your city and how it works in order to develop a project suited to local needs' (WHO 1995c: p15). Green (1992: p126) states that 'information is the lifeblood of the planning process. Without information it would be difficult to make any realistic decisions at all.' The information required is related to the previous discussion on the links between the environment (broadly defined) and health.

Selecting the information to be used in planning is not an objective process and the information available is not always useful. Politics are involved both in the choice of what information to collect, what information to use and the ways in which information is used. It is important for information to be as reliable, valid, current and understandable as possible. It is equally important to avoid the temptation of collecting data (much of which may be irrelevant to the planning process) ad nauseam as it is an expensive and time consuming process. For these reasons, the WHO has produced

Healthy City Projects in Developing Countries

guidelines related to the types of information that are required for healthy city projects to proceed (WHO 1995a). The guidelines promote a systematic interpretation of the types of information needed and by making the information gathering process explicit and consultative, political and other biases may be avoided.

The WHO guidelines (1995a) suggest that information gathering can be organized around ten questions (see Box 3.1). From this list of questions it can be seen that the types of information required for planning a healthy city vary considerably. Much of the information required is not health service related and frequently information refers to sectors other than health, for example, transport, industry, education or environment. This reinforces the intersectoral nature of healthy city projects and is a response to the recognition of the links between health status and environmental conditions discussed in the previous section. Each question in Box 3.1 will now be considered in turn and examples of the type of information referred to will be provided.

Box 3.1 Ten Questions around which Information can be Organized

1. What are the important health problems in the city?
2. How do economic and social conditions affect health?
3. Whose support is essential for project success?
4. How do city politics work?
5. How does the city administration function?
6. What are the concerns of the health care system?
7. What part do citizen groups play in city life?
8. How will national and regional programmes affect the project?
9. Will business, industry and labour support the project?
10. Where can information for project development be found?

Source: Adapted from WHO (1995a)

Important Health Problems in the City

Information is required on the mortality and morbidity associated with the major conditions of mental and physical ill health in the urban population. Health data can be either health service based or population based. Each type of data has its uses, for example, health service data will provide an indication of the types of problems staff are dealing with and is therefore useful for health service planning. Population based data on health problems will reveal the levels of suffering in a community providing information useful for deciding what intervention strategies to pursue. In certain cases, the burden of a particular disease in the community will not be reflected in a similar burden on the health services.

Equally important is information on whether or not some population groups (for example people living in a particular area, people from a particular ethnic group, people in a specific age group) suffer disproportionately from certain health problems. Basic demographic data, such as population distribution by age and geographical area, is therefore useful. The main causes of the important health problems should also be looked into and this aspect relates closely to the following section which elaborates on the economic and social conditions that affect health.

There has been some discussion about the possibility of using a relatively new technique for calculating the disease burden in developing country cities. The technique under discussion is the analysis of the burden of disease through the calculation of disability-adjusted life years (DALYs) as described by the World Bank (1993) and WHO (1996b). Although it is beyond the scope of this chapter to provide a detailed outline of the features of DALYs, the implications of a more widespread adoption of the techniques will be discussed briefly.

DALYs are calculated on the basis of various premises:

- that any health outcome representing loss of welfare should be included in indicators of health status;

- that the individual's characteristics considered in the calculations should be restricted to age and sex;
- that like health outcome should be treated as like; and
- that time is the unit of measurement (Murray 1994).

The use of DALYs in burden of disease analyses has been applauded by some due to their international comparability, the inclusion of data on both mortality and morbidity, and the relatively explicit valuation involved. However, various criticisms of the technique have been voiced, and Barker and Green (1996) provide a summary of the potential pitfalls in using the DALY approach:

- it espouses a limited view of health and health care due to the use of a single measure;
- it reinforces the medical model of health through focusing on single disease outcomes and interventions;
- it focuses on vertical disease-specific interventions;
- it lacks a consideration of lay people's values, all value judgements were made by 'experts';
- it is debatable whether the construction of DALYs at the local or national level in developing countries is a realistic option due to the expense involved.

From the above list it can be seen that many aspects of DALYs go against the main themes of healthy city projects. Burden of disease analyses have an implicit focus on vertical, frequently health service based, interventions of known efficacy whereas the ethos of healthy city projects is to follow an integrated route to health and one which involves changes in processes related to management, planning and community participation. A handful of *national* burden of disease analyses have been undertaken in developing countries (for example Mexico and Colombia), and other developing countries (for example South Africa) have attempted to initiate national burden of disease studies, but progress to date has been slow. It seems unlikely that, in the near future at least, city level burden of disease studies will be undertaken in developing countries due to their expense and need for specialist analysts. Within the context of healthy city projects, local burden of disease analyses are likely to be of limited value due to the reasons suggested at the beginning of this paragraph. However, international and regional burden of disease analyses may provide useful background information for urban health planners.

Economic and Social Conditions that Affect Health

As explained in the section on linking health status to environmental conditions, one of the key factors in healthy city projects is the recognition of the importance of economic and social conditions that affect health. Information related to the culture, religion, income distribution and employment opportunities in the city and how these relate to the local health situation described above, should be collected. This is obviously a broad and important part of the information needed for decision making related to health and requires input from a variety of actors.

Support Needed for Project Success

Healthy city projects cannot function without co-operation from a number of urban groups and actors. Support relates not only to financial resources, but also to political will, community organization and mobilization around health issues, the involvement (financial and otherwise) of local businesses and industry and backing from local NGOs (all discussed in more detail below). Without support from these different groups, it is unlikely that a healthy city project will fulfil its remit as a participatory, intersectoral, sustainable programme. It is therefore important that information is collected so that the availability of different kinds of support can be assessed and any gaps in support identified.

In addition, a healthy city project may not be a stand-alone project in a given city, it may be a health component of a larger urban development effort that involves urban infrastructure, land management, municipal finance, industrial development, etc, with the City Health Plan being an integral part of the wider development. Examples of such links include the joint Healthy City and

Sustainable City Program in Ibadan (where a City Health Plan is integrated into the development plan for the city) and the joint effort on healthy city projects and urban infrastructure development in several secondary towns in Bangladesh by the WHO and the Asian Development Bank. In such cases, it is important to have information on the support available from the link between the healthy city project and other urban development programmes so that efforts are not duplicated unnecessarily and so that a co-ordinated drive towards healthy urban development can be achieved.

Description of City Politics

Politics, as described later in this chapter, play a key role in the link between information gathering and priority setting. It is therefore crucial that those involved in setting up a healthy city project attempt to acquire an in depth understanding of how local politics function: how politicians are elected/appointed; who holds the most power; what is the status and tenure of the mayor; do the health sector and other health–environment issues feature in the current agenda; what is the community's role in the political process; and how autonomous is the local government from the regional and central governments. It is common for local government officials to play key roles in the development of a healthy city project: in such cases it is important for their influence in both spheres to be clearly defined.

Description of City Administration

Equally important is gaining an understanding of the structure and interrelationship of the different government departments along with the hierarchy and appointment procedure for administrative staff, particularly within the health department. A key issue for healthy city projects involves investigating whether environmental health is separated from health services delivery in the administration. Information related to the budget and how it is disbursed between departments (in particular looking at the share devoted to health and environment matters) will provide an insight into the status and priority accorded to different issues by the prevailing political powers.

Concerns of the Health Care System

Although the emphasis of healthy city projects is on the links between environmental conditions and health, health services still have an important role to play, (as discussed in Chapter 2) particularly in the provision of preventive and basic curative care. Analysing the distribution, type and use of health services available, along with their accessibility and acceptability to the local population is of interest. Current issues in the provision of health services should also be discovered.

Part Played by Citizen Groups in City Life

As previously mentioned, community participation is one of the key aspects of healthy city projects. Finding out whether communities are already organized and mobilized around health, environment or other related issues, how these groups function, who is involved in them and how they developed, will assist in later attempts to encourage further participation in relation to the project.

Description of National, Regional and International Programmes that might affect the Project

Knowledge of the existence and main activities of different national, regional and international programmes that may have an impact (positive or negative) on the healthy city project is important. Networking between such groups is a critical aspect of a project and one which is described later in this chapter. Before healthy city project actors become involved in new networking activities it is useful to discover the current networks that exist in relation to health and environmental issues in the cities. Identifying any potential obstacles to support for the project and the possible ways of overcoming them is an important step in the development of the project.

Potential for Support from Business, Industry and Labour for the Project

As mentioned above, support from local business, industry and labour is important for the ultimate success of a healthy city project. Identification of where such support readily exists and where it will need to be encouraged is required. The support can be of various types for example moral, financial and the provision of facilities or equipment.

Sources of Information for Project Development

Where will all the information for a healthy city project be found? In most developing country cities it is highly unlikely that there will be up-to-date accurate data related to all the categories mentioned. There are, however, likely to be a variety of useful documents with information related to the city of interest. The first stage in any information gathering exercise should involve discovering what relevant data already exists and in cases where existing data appears to be of adequate validity, subjecting it to rigorous analysis. Relevant data might, as previously suggested, be found in sectors other than health, for example, transport, education, environment, and it might also be related to a scale different from that at which priority setting will ultimately take place. Local government and university publications may prove useful sources of information. International, regional and national information might also be useful as might information collected at the district level. In addition to discovering what existing information is available, there is an opportunity to collect new information for the planning of a healthy city project. For example healthy city project consultants' reports may prove useful as would consultation with community members and local experts in both the public and private sectors. Methods for collecting new data are discussed below.

Methods of Gathering New Information

Broadly speaking, the methods used in health data collection can be divided into those that are quantitative in nature and those that are qualitative. The former represent what are largely traditional methods in the health field and the latter represent the more recent expansion of the social sciences into health (see Atkinson 1996 for a description of social research in health). Quantitative and qualitative data are both useful for health planning and it is important for health planners to understand the strengths and limitations of different types of data. In many instances, policy actors prefer making decisions on the basis of apparently 'scientific' quantitative information alone. This is mistaken as it has frequently been demonstrated that the use of such 'hard' statistics provides only a limited view of the complex processes that go towards creating the health profile of a particular population group. Qualitative, textual data has a lot to offer the urban health planner by providing a more in depth understanding of some of the processes involved and by considering the influence the socio-cultural context might have on urban health events. Qualitative methods of data collection are also particularly useful in healthy city projects where there is an explicit focus on community participation, changing the way key actors in the local government think about health and analysing local government processes, all topics that readily lend themselves to qualitative methods. Quantitative techniques are useful because they provide readily understandable data on, for example, death rates from various diseases. Table 3.1 provides a brief introduction to the various techniques involved for both quantitative and qualitative data collection and examples of ways in which they might be used in healthy city projects. The choice of method should always depend on the question being asked. It is for this reason that Table 3.1 begins with an outline of the types of question that qualitative and quantitative methods are designed to answer.

It should be remembered that qualitative and quantitative methods are inherently complementary: in many ways the weaknesses of one technique form the strengths of the other. The means by which information is collected to assist in the identification of priorities within the healthy city process should include relatively qualitative, participatory methods designed to elucidate the needs and priorities of the communities involved along with more quantitative, technical methods designed to provide an assessment based on available health statistics and show links between health status and environmental and social conditions (WHO 1996c). Aspects of the participatory process on the one hand and the technical data gathering and analysis on the other need to be reconciled through a consultative process (discussed in the section on priority setting). One way in which such reconciliation can take place is through the use of rapid appraisal techniques (see below), which are largely qualitative in nature, used in conjunction with survey techniques, which are quantitative in nature, designed to investigate the particular issues brought to light by the rapid appraisal.

Rapid Appraisal Techniques for Urban Areas

One method of data collection that has been successfully employed in a variety of settings including healthy city projects (for example in Campinas, Brazil) is rapid appraisal. The use of rapid appraisal techniques for analysing the health situation in a particular context sprang from the two approaches of rapid epidemiological assessment and rapid rural appraisal (with its origins in agricultural studies). Rapid appraisal for health is a relatively quick and cheap method for collecting information on the health situation in a particular community. The main features of rapid appraisal are that it: involves the community in the data collection process; has a multidisciplinary approach to data collection; focuses on achieving equity and empowerment by concentrating on those most in need; uses techniques that can be adapted to be appropriate to the local setting; and uses local knowledge (WHO 1988). Such features readily lend rapid appraisal techniques to the healthy city process as participatory information gathering can enhance community participation in other aspects of the project.

The specific methods involved in a rapid appraisal are the analysis of existing documents, conducting interviews with key informants on health and environment issues, and carrying out observations of the local area. Through this combination of techniques, rapid appraisals attempt to provide a broad picture of the health situation and one which takes community views fully into account.

Table 3.1 *Qualitative and Quantitative Methods*

	Qualitative	*Quantitative*
Types of questions answered	■ Exploratory ■ Explanatory	■ Descriptive ■ Explanatory
Main characteristics of method	■ Participatory, interactive ■ Informal ■ Small sample size ■ Intensive	■ Non-participatory ■ Formal ■ Large sample size ■ Extensive
Breakdown of methods	■ Focus group discussions ■ In depth interviews ■ Participant observation	■ Cohort study ■ Case-control study ■ Cross-sectional study (survey)
Type of data acquired	■ Textual	■ Statistical
Strengths of method	■ Contextualizes data ■ Provides in depth information	■ Generalizable ■ Accepted by policy makers
Weaknesses of method	■ Less accepted by policy makers ■ Less generalizable	■ De-contextualizes ■ Superficial ■ False claims of objectivity
Example of use related to health services	■ Focus groups with users of health services to discover ways in which they feel the service could be improved	■ Statistical analysis of health service records to discover main problems dealt with and their distribution through time
Example of use related to communities	■ Focus groups to discover community members' main health concerns and suggestions for tackling them	■ Household survey to collect information on recent health events and the type of help sought
Example of use related to local government	■ In depth interviews with key policy makers to investigate the extent to which health issues feature on their agendas	■ Cost benefit analysis of allocation of resources to different projects

Source: Blue (Work in progress)

The gathering of information during the early stages of a healthy city project has a direct link with the process of evaluation (see Chapter 4). The initial information gathered provides baseline data on which any changes (good or bad) can be measured. In Chapter 4 issues linked to some of those described above will be covered.

The ultimate aim of the information gathering process in healthy city projects is to produce a situation analysis that can inform priority setting. It should be remembered that the health situation in any city is dynamic. For this reason, the situation analysis should be reviewed on a regular basis, updated, and gaps in the data identified and, where possible, filled. The following section describes the way in which information gathering and the situation analysis are linked with priority setting.

PRIORITY SETTING

> 'Priorities are about change. Setting priorities to achieve best possible value for the resources available should be based on considerations of both benefits and costs. Using scarce resources in any way means, by definition, giving up the opportunity to use them in some other way; providing benefits here means forgoing them elsewhere. Priority setting means developing analyses and procedures to ensure that the policies that get priority (that is, those which get a higher call on extra resources) are the ones that provide the greatest benefits per additional dollar spent' (Mooney and Creese 1993: p731).

In an ideal situation the types of information described in Box 3.1 would be made available and key actors in the healthy city project would be able to produce a list of major problems. This list could then be prioritized through a process of open consultation with interested parties, including representatives from the local community. Once the problems have been prioritized possible solutions can be considered taking into consideration their cost and effectiveness which should include an examination of the local context. The list of priority solutions or actions would inform the creation of the City

Health Plan and allow resources (financial resources, community participation, etc) to be mobilized in ways most likely significantly to reduce the burden of ill health in the city. However, in reality there are various obstacles that act to prevent informed, explicit priority setting from taking place. The obstacles range from the relatively straightforward, for example insufficient funds or expertise available to collect the necessary information, to the more complex, for example the distribution of power and vested interests among key actors in the policy process.

A frequent misconception among public health researchers is that information will automatically feed into policy decisions. In fact it has been suggested that this is only rarely the case. Indeed, Hunt stated that

> 'By and large, policy makers seek to remedy current rather than future ills, many of which may be in-house rather than of significance to society at large, and work towards short-term rather than long-term goals. Decisions are rarely taken because of the evidence, rather evidence may be used to support existing positions and processes' (Hunt 1993: p71).

Hunt went on to say that 'Knowledge is translated into action only under particular sets of circumstances, many of the elements of which may be entirely fortuitous' (Hunt 1993: p73). Barker (1996) suggested that problems arise in the link between research and policy development because the policy development depends on factors beyond the control of those involved in information gathering. She commented that the legal environment, the level of commitment of officials to change and the level of support for change from other stakeholders are all important factors in the policy process. Walt (1994: p187) stated that 'Policy makers are only likely to use research results they find palatable, viable, persuasive or gratifying.' Clearly political processes are heavily involved in priority setting and decision making. The extent to which local politics lend themselves to open consultation and community involvement is of crucial importance to the decision-making process and the links between it and the information gathering process. Local people will only participate in action to solve particular problems if they feel it is important; community participation in the information gathering and priority setting process is thus vital for successful positive change to take place. It depends on a range of factors including the extent to which the local community is empowered and the transparency and levels of corruption in the prevailing political system.

The problems in the link between information gathering and priority setting can be divided into those problems that are related to the nature of the data (for example: poor quality data; old data; data not collected at an appropriate scale; and data not in a 'user friendly' format) and those related to the policy makers (for example: vested interests; suspicions regarding the quality of available data; unaccustomed to the use of data in decision making). The link between information gathering and priority setting might be enhanced if those involved in the data collection involve the policy makers and local community from the start allowing them to play a key role in identifying what information should be collected and, in certain circumstances, assisting in the data collection. In addition the information gathered should be presented in an accessible and understandable way to both policy makers and the community. Tackling the second set of issues related to policy makers is not as simple and calls for good governance.

The WHO Healthy City guidelines provide suggestions as to how strategic planning should proceed. For example, it is stated that some projects 'publish position statements that concentrate on the philosophy of the project and the health problems it considers to be priorities' (WHO 1995d: p32). However, little information is provided on how such priorities are to be identified. *'Building a healthy city: a practitioner's guide, a step-by-step approach to implementing healthy city projects in low-income countries'* produced by the WHO (WHO 1995a) also provides much useful information on how to set up healthy city projects and what types of information can be useful for decision making, but one of its weakest elements relates to its guidance on the process of prioritization. This is not surprising when it is considered that in health literature in general, the process of prioritization, although considered one of the most difficult and important stages in the planning process, has received relatively little attention (Green 1992).

Although the healthy city literature provides relatively little insight into the process of priority setting, it does emphasize *who* should be involved in problem identification and priority setting. The need for intersectoral collaboration is stressed as is the need for representatives from different organizations: local government, NGOs, university staff, private enterprises. Perhaps the main point to be gained from the healthy city literature is the need for community or citizen participation in the formation of a multisectoral City Health Plan. The issue of community participation in healthy city projects is topical (Petersen 1996) and is something that forms an integral part of the healthy city philosophy. Advocating community participation in identifying local health needs and establishing priority areas for action is one thing, achieving it is another. In industrialized countries draft City Health Plans have been sent out to the community for a period of consultation. For example, in the Liverpool Healthy City (UK) a summary guide to the draft Liverpool City Health Plan with a short questionnaire attached was sent out to inhabitants. Respondents were asked for their opinion of the plan and they were provided with the opportunity to comment on the plan and suggest ways in which it could be altered. In most developing country cities, however, the prevalence of illiteracy would seriously affect the representativeness and ultimate usefulness of such a procedure. The WHO manual (WHO 1995d) suggests that:

'Helping communities to assess their needs and preferences provides the groundwork for participation. Frequently their view of what is needed differs from those of professionals and people working within city departments. An effective approach is to provide financial and technical support while allowing community groups to design and carry out the necessary survey of needs in their area' (WHO 1995d: p44).

Apart from WHO guidance as to who should be involved in setting priorities for healthy city projects it is possible to draw out other information on prioritization from existing literature and experience to date. Prioritization takes place at different stages during the healthy city process: prioritizing what new information to gather; prioritization among task forces; and prioritization at the steering committee level. Each will be considered in turn.

Prioritizing what New Information to Gather

Identifying gaps in the available information related to healthy city projects is a subjective process. Different people with different perspectives on health and how it is gained and maintained will have different views on the type of information required before appropriate prioritization can take place. For this reason, any suggestions for new, specific research studies to be carried out within the framework of a healthy city project should be accompanied by a clear justification of the need for such a study which can then be reviewed by the steering committee. Collecting information costs money and takes time and should not be undertaken haphazardly.

Prioritizing among Task Forces (Working Groups)

In healthy city projects task forces are created so that small groups of people can pursue particular areas of concern in detail. However, the decision as to what task forces should be set up is clearly of importance and should be based on a preliminary assessment of local needs. In general (as explained in Chapter 2) there should be task forces to cover the major aspects of the urban environment that affect health, for example: water, sanitation, health services, education, transport, industry, socio-cultural affairs. Members of the task force can include local experts in that area, but also community members and other interested parties.

Each task force should identify the problems within that particular sector that have an impact on health. The issues can be identified from the situation analysis and also from additional information provided and collected by those in the task force. Participation from community members in problem identification should be sought. The list of problems can then be reviewed and ranked according to their priority in terms of their negative impact on health. It is important that both current and expected problems be taken into consideration. The process of ranking is key and requires the formulation of a consensus. A consensus can be reached through a variety of means, but usually involves a workshop run by a facilitator who should aim to ensure everyone participates. Members can express their views verbally or anonymously in writing (which is often useful in situations where very powerful and less powerful people are members of the same task force, but may not be feasible if any members are illiterate).

Once a ranked list of problems has been produced, the ways in which the problems can be solved should be considered. Where financial resources are limited, priority should go to those solutions that can reduce the health burden the most, at the lowest cost and with the highest chances of success, given the local circumstances and opportunities for exploiting non-financial resources such as human capital, existing infrastructure and community involvement. This calls for consideration of community perceptions of the issues, as people will only act on problems they consider to be of importance. Many of these decisions are difficult to make and even in situations where detailed information *is* available on the cost-effectiveness of various interventions, such decisions rely on value judgements. In situations where information on cost-effectiveness of interventions is severely limited it is likely that value judgements will play an even greater role. Because of the origins of the members of the different task forces (comprising local government officials, academics, community members, technical experts, etc), consensus building is likely to produce inherently different results than if the task forces had been formed of, for example, only medical professionals or members of the local government. This is one of the key ways in which healthy city projects differ from traditional health planning.

Prioritizing at the Level of the Steering Committee

The priorities identified by the task forces are reviewed by the steering committee which is responsible for identifying overall city-wide priorities within the framework of existing local and national resources. It is at this stage that an overall City Health Plan can be developed, incorporating the issues raised by the various task forces. The City Health Plan should include information on priority actions and programmes including the setting of targets and plans for evaluation (see Chapter 4).

Once priorities have been set it should be possible to write a City Health Plan which will include information on the main activities that will form part of the project (see Box 2.2 for an outline of a City Health Plan. The responsibilities of different actors in implementing the activities need to be made clear as do the resources to be mobilized, the deadline for completion and the ultimate aim of each activity (see Table 2.1, p30, for an example from Chittagong).

ACTION

Because of the city-specific nature of healthy city projects it is impossible to draw up a comprehensive list of activities that would be undertaken. However, one component of the City Health Plan invariably includes matters related to enhancing local participation in the project through reports in the local media and campaigns on particular issues. In addition, networking at various levels is a key activity for all healthy city projects and is considered in some detail below. This is followed by a discussion of a popular approach to activities, namely the 'settings' approach. This differs from a more traditional organization of activities around topics or administrative units. The chapter ends with a consideration of the implementation of healthy city projects in three case studies. In this way it is hoped that the reader will gain further insight into the processes that have been described above.

Networking

In some countries, it has been helpful to establish a 'National Healthy Cities Commission', or network, and each project city may serve as a model for other cities. A clear commitment by such a body to local government policies that reduce marginalization or exclusion of poor communities from socio-economic life and services can greatly assist local efforts.

In addition, the WHO actively promotes the healthy city approach worldwide. The WHO organizes inter-country meetings in all regions on a regular basis, to review the progress of the participating cities, and for exchange of health and environmental technologies, and experiences with successful projects. Participating cities have their project co-ordinator entered into an international database, and newsletters and technical reports are regularly circulated. Potential project co-ordinators and supporters are encouraged to contact and seek support from the global, regional or, in some cases, national networks of healthy cities. City to city level contacts are well known as major routes of exchange of information, technology, commerce and trade, etc, and have now assumed importance in the area of health. The phenomenon of 'city twinning' where a closer relationship is established between cities that have particular ties based on culture, language, shared historical events or other bonds, has become commonplace. City networking for health can draw on these links, but does so in a purposeful way to develop a shared agenda to improve health and environment conditions. Important networks have developed by language, for instance the Francophone and Spanish speaking networks of healthy city projects. Examples of networking include:

- established healthy cities assist cities developing new projects, during the 'start-up' phase of their projects;
- multi-city action plans (MCAPs); this approach has become very popular in some regions, for example, Europe, and involves a number of healthy cities that decide simultaneously to address a particular health issue, such as alcohol, nutrition, AIDS, diabetes, women's health, etc. Cities agree that their situation analyses, approaches and strategies, programmes and monitoring data will be shared in the implementation of the plan and programme. In

this way the resources of many cities are brought to bear on the issue in each participating city;
- exchange of experiences of healthy city projects in organized national, regional and global networking activities.

Many other activities designed to improve the capacity of municipal government to manage the urban environment and improve living conditions in cities have taken place in the wake of UNCED. In addition to the WHO Healthy City Project and UNDP's LIFE Programme, the UNDP/World Bank/UNCHS' (United Nations Centre for Human Settlements') Urban Management Programme, the ILO's (International Labour Office's) Labour Intensive Public Works Programme, the Metropolitan Environment Improvement Programme and Metropolitan Development Programme of the World Bank/UNDP, the Sustainable Cities Programme of UNCHS, the CITYNET/Asia-Pacific 2000 Programme of ESCAP (Economic and Social Committee of Asia and the Pacific)/UNDP, the Megacities Programme, the Metropolis Programme, and various international organizations concerned with local government, are major initiatives at the international level.

The Settings Approach

This approach has become popular in healthy city projects. Settings are major structures that provide channels and mechanisms of influence for reaching defined populations. The city as a whole may be viewed as a setting. Background information on the settings approach was provided in Chapter 1 and Box 1.3 (see p17) outlined some of its main features.

The use of the settings approach in healthy city projects involves focusing activities on a particular setting, for example healthy villages, healthy schools, healthy workplaces, healthy food markets, health promoting hospitals with the following characteristics: (adapted from WHO 1995a).

Schools

Schools in the city may participate in a 'healthy schools' project that addresses parental and teacher involvement, and child participation in relevant school management and decision making. There may be projects to improve water facilities, toilets, school playgrounds and classrooms. Environment and health education can be strengthened with grade-appropriate curricula. There should also be attention to a school medical service that emphasizes prevention.

Workplaces

A 'healthy and safe workplace' programme would necessarily operate on two levels: the 'traditional' occupational health service that emphasizes factory level work by health inspectors, and the newer challenge of the SSI which demands community-based and participatory approaches.

There are many important issues. For example: the education of workers about matters such as assessing risks and understanding safe procedures; support and training within NGOs related to the education of workers in SSIs; worker participation and representation in industry management and industry/trade associations; the involvement of the mass media in education; the provision of health services for workers; attention to the needs of women workers and support for women's associations; establishing channels of communication between managers, workers and authorities responsible for environmental protection; proper management of solid and liquid wastes; and siting industries in locations that reduce pollution and environmental damage.

Market Places

A 'healthy market places' programme establishes partnerships between all concerned to address issues such as the health conditions of stall-holders and food handlers (water, toilets, availability of health services); how foodstuffs are handled and stored; how to minimize any adverse impacts of markets on surrounding residential areas; garbage removal and maintenance of cleanliness of the market area; the methods of inspection by government authorities (for example, how food inspectors can play a more educational rather than a punitive role); and finally the role of the market place in health education.

Health Centres and Hospitals

Important areas for consideration in a 'health services upgrade' are the development of inputs from the user community to the decision-making processes and management of the health centres; the strengthening and promotion of preventive services alongside curative services; and greater equity in provision.

Partnerships may form between women's organizations, health-oriented NGOs, and ministry of health and municipal health agencies responsible for provision of health services, or for running health centres or managing hospitals, to address local priority issues. For example: how to make maternal–child health services more accessible for under-served areas; improved family planning; improved health education; better and more appropriate and readily available drug therapies for common diseases, etc.

The settings approach has been adopted in various cities, but it is not the only way for activities in a healthy city project to be structured. Those involved in different settings need to be made aware of activities in other settings so that duplication of efforts is avoided and cross-setting issues are addressed in a co-ordinated manner.

CASE STUDIES

As healthy city projects in developing countries are still relatively young, there are only a few that have been through the process of priority setting and proceeded towards implementing the City Health Plan. What follows is a description of how implementation has proceeded in three case studies, Fayoum in Egypt, Quetta in Pakistan and Campinas in Brazil. Some additional information is also provided on a number of other cities.

CASE STUDY: FAYOUM, EGYPT

The Fayoum Governorate is a natural depression situated approximately 90 km from Cairo. The area has a rich history with many ancient sites from Pharaonic, Graeco–Roman and Islamic civilization. Fayoum is a densely populated region of closely packed villages and towns with around 2 million inhabitants. The main economic activities are related to agricultural production. Many health indicators (for example, infant and child mortality rates, immunization coverage, population per health care unit) compare unfavourably with national averages and Fayoum has various problems related to basic infrastructure, and health and social service provision.

The Healthy City Project in Fayoum began in 1995 with a workshop at which key local policy makers presented their views on how activities in their sector influenced health, and the main problems they felt needed to be addressed (Harpham and Blue 1995). Local elected leaders were also asked to attend the workshop and they contributed to the discussions on the major health problems in the area. It was decided to focus initially on three specific sites in the hope that healthy city project activities would then spread to other sites. Following this, existing data related to the city and country was collected and semi-structured interviews were held with key policy makers, hospital and health centre staff, and local leaders (including the leaders of women's groups). Focus group discussions were held with staff at various health centres, and health centre and hospital records were analysed. In addition, a brief questionnaire was conducted among local women seeking to understand their health needs and priorities. In settings where community participation, even in the smallest capacity, is in no way routine it is important to emphasize the need to involve local people in the various stages of the project; information gathering, problem identification, priority setting.

On the basis of the information collected and analysed, a preliminary situation analysis was produced (Harpham and Blue 1995). A list of the priorities mentioned by those who participated in the fieldwork was included in the report, this is reproduced as Box 3.2 (they are not in order of priority).

Healthy City Projects in Developing Countries

> **Box 3.2 Priority Areas in Fayoum, Egypt**
>
> - Health and housing: good design for a house, cleanliness inside the home; control of rodents; overcrowding; ventilation.
> - Income generation: provision of low-interest loans.
> - Sanitation: sewerage system; emptying of septic tanks.
> - Food safety in the home and market place.
> - Healthy animal husbandry: separate animal and human living quarters; hygiene at slaughterhouse.
> - Women's community participation: decrease illiteracy; reduce female circumcision; decrease occurrence of early marriage.
> - Youth action on health: promote youth centres.
> - Healthy schools: fibre glass water storage tanks; maintenance and rehabilitation of latrines; improve health insurance; tackle anaemia and malnutrition; reduce class density.
> - Health and safety at work: problem of pesticides and herbicides being applied by hand.
> - Water: rising of subsoil water; water pollution; shortage of water.
> - Land use planning, zoning: to prevent desertification.
> - Health and hygiene education: creation of public washing places; literacy classes.
> - Health centres: need vehicles; communication with hospital, lack basic drugs; need better equipment.
>
> Source: Harpham and Blue (1995)

From this list it can be seen that healthy city projects can address a wide range of problem areas and require inputs from many sectors in the local government, private sector and community. Indeed, only one point on the list focused explicitly on health services. Following the production of the above mentioned report, a second workshop was held in February 1996 and the steering committee decided to select six issues to be tackled first, given available resources: healthy schools; water supply; health and hygiene education; garbage removal and disposal; drainage and sanitation; and income generation. A 1995/96 Plan of Action was drawn up and it was decided to focus energy on addressing two issues, healthy schools and on-site sanitation. The Plan of Action included details of what was to be done, by whom, with what deadline, for what purpose and with what resources. Implementation of the Plan has been quite successful although some aspects still need to be addressed. There has been progress in carrying out a needs assessment of the water, sanitation and solid waste facilities in schools, and school staff have been trained in health and hygiene issues. In addition surveys have been conducted of on-site sanitation facilities, but progress in this aspect has been limited due to lack of funds.

A second Plan of Action incorporating the 1995/96 Plan was devised for 1996/97 and in this four issues were identified: health education and promotion; water and waste water; environmental sanitation; and income generation (Werna 1997). Working groups were created to address each of the issues. Substantial progress has been made in all four components of the Plan although much of this is due to the keen support provided by the local government. In the future it will be important for the Healthy City Project to seek greater participation from the community, local stakeholders and other potential funders (Werna 1997).

CASE STUDY: QUETTA, PAKISTAN

The Quetta Healthy City Project began in 1995 (see Chapter 2 for further background information on this Project). During the start-up phase a consultant's report was prepared (Werna 1995b). The report consisted of a review of the healthy city process, a situation analysis, a list of existing gaps in data and recommendations for action. It was suggested that the following gaps in data needed to be filled: urban development and health for Pakistan, Balochistan and Quetta; the main preventable causes of death in Quetta; housing and health; refugees and migrants; occupational health; education and health conditions in schools; health services; urban informal sector; and future development options. In addition, the report listed priorities for action based on the preliminary information collected from discussions with local institutions and from a limited number of reports (see Box 3.3). The list is not in order of priority. It was suggested that the list be reviewed and elaborated upon by the task forces during the preparation of the City Health Plan.

Healthy City Projects in Developing Countries

> **Box 3.3 Initial List of Priorities for Quetta Healthy City Project**
>
> - Governance and institutional integration
> - Land development and housing
> - Economic development and healthy workplaces
> - Socio-cultural issues
> - Water
> - Sanitation and sewerage
> - Drainage
> - Solid waste
> - Roads, traffic and transportation
> - Energy
> - Environmental protection
> - Education and healthy schools
> - Health services
> - Funding opportunities for Quetta Healthy City Project
>
> Source: Werna (1995)

The next consultant's report (Werna 1996b) reviewed the start-up phase and made preparations for the organization phase of the Project. It was suggested that a Quetta Profile be prepared 'providing information on the various sectors of activity in the city (for example housing, water, education), their impacts on health, and an inventory of the organizations and resources in each sector'. The link between the Profile and the Quetta Healthy City Plan of Action was stressed. Following on from the 14 priority areas identified during the start-up phase of the Project, task forces were developed. The task forces were constituted in such a way so as to encompass all the aspects of urban health and development previously identified. The final choice of task groups was decided upon after a phase of broad consultation within the steering group and with representatives from local organizations. The seven Quetta Healthy City task forces (environmental health services; housing and land devilment; roads, transport and energy; economic development; education; social affairs; health services) were discussed in Chapter 2.

The task forces were formed during a workshop in 1996. They were asked to identify the main problems in their area and make suggestions as

Implementing Healthy City Projects

to how the problems could be addressed. This exercise will feed directly into the preparation of the Quetta Healthy City Plan of Action. In addition to the seven main areas of activity, it was suggested that three initial projects should be developed: an environmental health project in one ward; a basic minimum needs project in another ward and a city-wide project (for example, curbing air pollution). The idea behind such pioneer projects is that it helps focus healthy city participants on particular activities while the bulk of the project revolves around planning in the early stages. Implementing small projects at the outset of the healthy city is also a way of increasing community awareness and motivation.

By May 1997 progress in the Quetta Healthy City Project had been limited mainly due to changes in national, provincial and local government and a change in project co-ordinator. Although some progress had been made in respect to information gathering, a health and environment profile of Quetta had not been compiled and as the Plan of Action depends upon the information in the profile document, it had not been devised (Harpham 1997). In addition, the task forces created in 1996 had ceased to function effectively. It is to be hoped that now there is a new project co-ordinator in place and a relatively stable political situation, further progress will be made.

CASE STUDY: CAMPINAS, BRAZIL

With a population of around 1 million, Campinas is the second largest city in the State of São Paulo, situated in the south-east of Brazil. São Paulo is the richest and most populous state in Brazil and Campinas plays an important role in the state's industrial, commercial and educational activities. Despite its relative economic success, Campinas displays the intra-urban differentials common throughout Brazil and there are approximately 182 slum areas (*favelas*) found mainly in the peripheral areas of the city with an estimated 10 per cent of the total population. The population growth rate in the *favelas* is almost three times the average for Campinas and the usual problems related to the physical and social environment found in such areas abound.

A healthy city project was initiated in Campinas towards the end of 1994 with an agreement between the municipal authorities and the WHO.

Campinas is divided into four administrative areas, each with an administrator accountable to the mayor. The Healthy City Project actors opted for a zonal rather than a sectoral approach and used the existing divisions as the basis for organization. Although action plans were drawn up for all four areas, it was decided to concentrate healthy city activities in just one of these administrative areas, namely SAR-NORTE (the northern area), in the hope that activities once established there, would eventually spread to the other areas. Within SAR-NORTE, the district of São Marcos (with a total population of 22,000) was chosen as the focus of the Healthy City Project as it was considered one of the most needy areas. A group consisting of local municipal officers, health advisers, representatives from local schools and representatives from the housing associations of the *favelas* was formed. Following this a rapid appraisal was carried out using interviews with key informants, analysis of existing documents and observation. The information collected was then presented at a workshop attended by approximately 450 people including the key informants, advisers, members of local NGOs, municipal officers and the mayor. From all the problems discussed, it was decided to focus on two particular issues: children and adolescents living on the streets; and the lack of infrastructure and sanitation in the *favelas*.

For each of the two problems, a list of causes and possible solutions were developed. In the case of children and adolescents living on the streets, local parents were asked to talk about their understanding of the problems. The main problem discussed was children and youths not attending schools and ending up on the streets. The main causes were cited as being: violence within the home, a lack of family structure; low levels of family income; a lack of appropriate training for adolescents; a lack of crèches and nursery schools; a lack of focus on community issues in school curricula; lack of a mental health and youth programme; and a lack of leisure opportunities. The possible solutions were linked to specific causes of the problem and included: implementing a programme directed to family relations; implementing a programme for managing income; devising a programme for schools; and creating areas for play and leisure activities.

In the case of the lack of infrastructure and sanitation, it was found that a large majority of people living in the *favelas* did not have sanitation facilities or rubbish collection. They lived in precarious settings that were often severely affected by flooding. In addition there were several lakes that were heavily polluted and contaminated with schistosomiasis. The main causes of the problems cited were: the haphazard occupation of the land; a lack of

> environmental education; and a lack of sanitation of the lakes. Solutions suggested included: providing infrastructure for *favelas*; relocating some families to new, planned settlements; implementing environmental education programmes; creating community environmental groups to replant trees and oversee environmental aspects of the community; and cleaning the lakes.
>
> At present many of the above mentioned solutions are in the process of being implemented in São Marcos. However, the original intention of spreading the Healthy City Project from São Marcos has yet to be fulfilled and appears to have been delayed due to recent changes in the municipal administration. (This issue will be further discussed in Chapter 6).

Examples from other Cities

In Managua, Nicaragua, where a healthy city project began in 1995, the gathering of additional information was to be undertaken by the local government. It was agreed that sector profiles should be compiled in the following areas; history of urban development, socio-economic factors, urban environment, infrastructure, production and industrial development, culture, education and health (Barten 1996). The information collected would then be used in the decision-making process surrounding the formulation of the City Health Plan.

In Accra, Ghana, where a healthy city project began in 1992, the initial meeting divided participants (local government officials, representatives from the private sector, media representatives, members of NGOs and representatives from community groups) into groups to examine the following problem areas: environmental sanitation, waste management and food hygiene; health problems and health service coverage; public education and communication in health; community involvement in health and sanitation; and planning and land use. The five areas were selected through plenary discussions and consensus. Following the first meeting a four-day workshop was held during which action plans were formed for the following three areas: environmental sanitation, waste management and urban planning; health problems, health service coverage and school health programmes; and education, communication and community involvement in sanitation and health. All action plans had to include a problem statement, objectives, strategies, activities, timing, persons responsible and resources needed (Blankers 1993)**. Box 3.4 provides further examples of healthy city project activities.

Box 3.4 Examples of Healthy City Project Activities

> In Tehran the Healthy City Project has led to an upgrading of housing in low income areas of the city.
>
> In Lahore the Project has focused on improving environmental and sanitary conditions in crowded informal settlements, using a partnership between the city corporation, local residents and other agencies.
>
> The Healthy City Project in Rio de Janeiro has mobilized the human and financial resources to provide drainage for a neighbourhood, stopping the seasonal flooding of low-lying areas.
>
> Healthy City partners in Chittagong have agreed on a programme of action covering seven main areas: slum improvement, literacy, water and sanitation, drainage and sewerage, health care and nutrition, and town planning.
>
> In Johannesburg the Healthy City Project has developed a comprehensive health and housing programme for townships in the vicinity of the city, with improvements already achieved in such areas as water, sanitation, solid waste management and neighbourhood safety.
>
> Source: Adapted from WHO (1995a: p14)

CONCLUSION

Ultimately, the processes of linking health status to environmental conditions, information gathering, priority setting, action and the production of a City Health Plan is a balancing act that requires the skills, knowledge and understanding of a variety of actors. The

---

** Eventually the Accra Project decided to concentrate on schools

participatory nature of information gathering and priority setting within healthy city projects and the inherently intersectoral focus should result in fundamentally different priorities than those that would have been reached had traditional, unintegrated, non-participatory techniques been employed. What each city prioritizes will depend not only on the local situation and the local ability to deal with that situation, but also national, regional and international factors that cannot be ignored.

The case studies demonstrate the variety of activities that can be involved in a healthy city project. Although similar *processes* are involved in all healthy city projects (community participation, intersectoral collaboration, city-level consultation, etc), each one comprises context-specific actions. Progress in healthy city projects is dependent on many factors, often political, and the range in the time taken to achieve certain steps in the projects described above demonstrates this.

4 Evaluating Healthy City Projects

Due to the early stage of development of healthy city projects in developing countries, there are few evaluations to date, some of which were mentioned in Chapter 2. However, it is possible to identify key issues in such evaluations and to provide some directions for future evaluations. All evaluations depend on good baseline data collected at the beginning of the project. Thus, this chapter is a natural follow on from the previous chapter which considered the information which is needed to design a healthy city project from the outset. As current healthy city initiatives are partly dependent on international aid agencies (for example, the Dutch bilateral donor) it is inevitable that effective evaluations of such projects will be required. Although evaluations are often seen as an end-of-project activity it is important to plan them from the beginning of a healthy city project and to ensure that any data used for regular monitoring purposes feeds into a final evaluation.

ISSUES AND DEFINITIONS IN EVALUATION

The late 1980s and 1990s have witnessed much debate on how to make evaluations in the field of international public health. Some of the discussions have been fuelled by the introduction of the idea of measuring the 'burden of disease' which was briefly covered in Chapter 3. It is possible to distil the following issues from the debate:

- getting the right balance between quantitative and qualitative methods;
- choosing the most appropriate indicators (particularly the debate between process and impact indicators, see Schrettenbrunner and Harpham 1993);
- the desirability of participatory, or bottom-up evaluations;
- the cost of evaluations vis-à-vis the total cost of project or programme implementation;
- increasing the use of project (or logical) frameworks which force the clear identification of inputs, activities, outputs, purpose and goal (see, for example, ODA 1995).

Evaluation of healthy city projects or programmes is not immune from these issues. However, the nature of the initiative means that particular subjects have to be addressed in this chapter:

(1) the emphasis on interaction with communities means that special attention must be paid to participatory evaluation;
(2) the limited emphasis on health service/sector action alone and the desire to include the activities of other sectors raises questions about the appropriateness of health impact indicators, and the duration and objectives of healthy city projects highlight the need for the use of process indicators;
(3) the involvement of international agencies (for example, bilateral agencies in a funding role and the WHO in a technical assistance role) raises issues about the use of locally generated versus internationally comparable indicators;
(4) the multitude of actors involved raises the question of relative vested interests and values in evaluations.

Before turning to these topics it is important to consider the definition and elements of evaluation. There is a sea of literature on evaluation, and, as Elzinger (1981) puts it, a veritable industry of activities connected with it. Although many definitions of evaluation can be found, the definition proposed by the UN is used throughout this chapter. Thus evaluation is a process which attempts to determine, as systematically and objectively as possible, the relevance, adequacy, effectiveness, efficiency and/or impact of activities in the light of predetermined objectives (WHO 1981). In the context of project evaluation, the following elements can be defined:

- *Inputs*. The set of means (money, equipment, materials, technical advice, training, etc) mobilized to produce the planned outputs.
- *Process*. The array of activities displayed by the project and the project's interaction with the community (for example, planning systems, management systems, training programmes).
- *Outputs*. The product of the system, which is often a service, such as staff time made available to the community, number of drains built, number of campaigns mounted.
- *Outcomes*. The effects (potent vaccines delivered to children of correct age, knowledge conveyed to communities at village meetings and so on) and coverage (percentages of eligible couples using contraception, attendance at antenatal care) of the outputs.
- *Impact*. Changes in morbidity, mortality, nutritional status or fertility (such as infant mortality rates). Confusingly, this definition is often given to the term 'outcome' in some literature.

The remainder of this chapter considers the issues identified above. Unlike the previous chapters, it does not include illustrative case studies from selected cities. This is because, as stated in the introductory chapter, the implementation of healthy city projects in developing countries is at an early stage, and few comprehensive evaluations have been undertaken to date. This chapter therefore serves as a guide for the design of future evaluations. The first issue to be covered is the participatory nature of evaluations. The debates about impact and process indicators and local versus international indicators are then considered followed by a discussion of values in evaluation and a conclusion which refers to the latest thinking about evaluating healthy city projects in developing countries.

COMMUNITY PARTICIPATION AND EVALUATION

Smithies and Adams (1993) argue that community participation strategies of the healthy city approach pose difficulties when it comes to evaluation for a number of reasons. First, there may be conflict between actors; second, the projects are developmental and outcomes are unpredictable; third, change takes place constantly; fourth, process is integral to healthy city projects and needs evaluation as much as any impact; and finally, evaluation methods should mirror the principles of the approach itself. 'What is needed is research and evaluation that focuses on illuminating the why and the how, as well as what and how many' (Smithies and Adams 1993: p59). The authors go on to argue that, in industrialized countries, there has been a bias towards complex, costly and highly quantitative evaluation methods which have neglected participatory principles. After presenting two case studies of participatory evaluation the authors argue for future evaluation and research on healthy city projects to embrace the principles of the new public health movement (see Ashton and Seymour (1988) *The New Public Health*).

One of the best participatory evaluations of a healthy city project appears to be that undertaken by Baum (1993a) in Noarlunga in Australia. This evaluation collected healthy city project information on:

- policy changes;
- collaboration between different sectors in services provision and planning;
- planning;
- community involvement and awareness;
- changes in the way local public service workers approached their work;
- key stakeholders' perceptions of the project.

The various methods used were:

- key informant interviews during the early stages of the project, then again at a later stage;
- audit of attendance at meetings of committee members;
- questionnaire surveys of key groups including management committee members, local health workers and the local community;
- analysis of local media;
- documentation of additional resources attracted to the activity;
- on-going monitoring of the project by members of the research team who played a role in the Healthy City Project.

Baum emphasizes that their evaluation encouraged critical appraisal of the developing Healthy City Project and that there is a danger, common to many new projects, that those involved with them become so immersed that they lose their perspective of the endeavour. The regularity of evaluation reports allowed time for assessment and reflection on the project's progress, which was particularly valued by the team. This is an argument for evaluations to be conducted by insiders rather than by outsiders, ie so-called independent evaluations. However, this is an issue which needs to be determined at the earliest stage of a healthy city project. All evaluations of healthy city projects should decide the extent to which the procedure is going to be participatory, at the outset. The more participatory the evaluation, the more useful are classic texts on participatory evaluation (for example, Feuerstein 1986). The ability of the community to participate in an evaluation may partly depend on the type of indicators used in the evaluation and this is discussed in the next section.

IMPACT AND PROCESS INDICATORS

Werna and Harpham (1995) summarize four different positions in the literature regarding the use of process and/or impact indicators for healthy city projects:

(1) the sole use of process indicators (for example, Blankers 1993; Davies and Kelly 1993; de Leeuw and Goumans 1993);
(2) the primary use of process indicators supplemented by a few impact indicators (for example, Baum 1993b);
(3) parallel use of both types of indicators (Draper et al 1993; WHO 1995d);
(4) the sole use of impact indicators (Collin 1992; WHO 1990).

However, none of these authors discussed the reasons for their choice of impact and/or process indicators. The authors who mention methodological issues concentrate on the debate between locally generated versus internationally generated indicators. Such a debate will be analysed in the next section. First, the specific use of impact and process indicators will be considered.

Impact and process indicators may be used together. However, it is usually appropriate to measure impact only after some years of intervention (for example, indicators such as infant mortality rate, prevalence of malaria, maternal death rate, atmospheric pollution, water quality, extent of green spaces). Although one could argue that long-term impact is what really matters, it is also important to assess the earliest years of healthy city projects in order to keep the morale of the participating actors high (by demonstrating progress and/or to correct potential problems). Donor agencies may also be willing to monitor the development of the project from the early stages. For instance, on the one hand, the Dutch bilateral donor agency, criticized a WHO request for funding healthy city projects in five developing countries in 1994 because their proposed evaluation was largely based on impact (long-term) indicators. On the other hand the WHO (1997a) has recently stressed that evaluations must provide the evidence needed to show what healthy city projects can do to improve health determinants (thus emphasizing impact measures).

Therefore, there is a need for medium, or even short-term, evaluation (often called formative evaluation). A number of impact indicators can be used in such an evaluation if within a healthy city project there is a pilot project – especially environmental indicators (such as water and sewerage provision, water quality, waste collection, extent of green space, public transport, living space), and socio-economic indicators (such as unemployment, homelessness, illiteracy). Pilot projects might play a symbolic role for example, the concentration of efforts to improve one specific squatter settlement or one ward in a city is likely to bring physical/visible results quickly, which in turn may motivate the population and institutions to continue supporting healthy city projects. However, pilot projects have been extensively criticized for not being sustainable and/or replicable and they also contradict the broad/holistic approach of the healthy city approach. Thus, impact indicators derived from pilot projects are unlikely to have significance for the city as a whole.

Considering the need for mid- or even short-term evaluation on the one hand, and the problems of using impact indicators on the other, process indicators assume a significant role in healthy city projects. Process indicators which assess issues such as level of community organization, awareness and participation of different actors or co-operation between participating institutions, are able to spot changes much quicker. It has recently been argued (WHO 1997a) that it is important to evaluate whether health has been placed high on the social and political agenda as a result of a healthy city project. This will reflect the effectiveness of key actors, particularly the co-ordinator.

In addition to the above points, process evaluations, especially those focusing on institution strengthening and capacity building, are important in assessing sustainability (see Chapter 5). It is possible to achieve improvements in health, environmental and socio-economic conditions in a given city via inputs from external actors, for instance via international or federal programmes. However, when such programmes come to an end, the improvements are likely to cease if local actors have not been prepared to carry them on. Therefore, it is fundamental to assess the capacities of local actors.

The importance of institution strengthening and capacity building has been highlighted in the guidelines for healthy city projects (WHO 1995a) as well as in the guidelines of other UN agencies' urban agendas and programmes. After decades of investing in specific projects, by the mid-1980s the UN agencies most active in the urban field shifted their focus from a 'project approach' to a 'process approach'. The new approach has entailed a focus on holistic/long-term processes of urban development, which are likely to generate more profound and sustainable results. Emphasis is given to the training and co-ordination of, and co-operation between, local actors which have been regarded as fundamental to the good management of a sustainable urban development process. These facts reinforce the importance of using process evaluation in healthy city projects.

Table 4.1 shows a range of indicators for evaluations of healthy city projects as proposed by the WHO. Some of what they term pressure indicators would be regarded by some as impact indicators (for example, death rates). The WHO usefully separates process and impact indicators and indicators of capacity development and community participation. Most impact indicators require measurement of health status and these call for epidemiological methods. Process indicators can be measured by qualitative methods, for example, interviews with key actors. Thus, a mix of methods is needed.

Regarding the debate on impact and process indicators, Harrison (1996) points out that if rigorous impact evaluation is attempted the construction of alternative scenarios in which both environmental and health outputs in the absence of a healthy city project would have to be forecasted. The additional impact of the healthy city project on such outputs could then be calculated. Most people would agree that this approach would be inappropriate and expensive although, as Harrison points out, there is no reason why healthy city projects should be immune to impact evaluations. Harrison goes on to suggest that insofar as healthy city projects are genuinely consensual and command local support across different interests, and do not make major claims on public expenditure and are therefore not expected to prove value for money, then it could be said that evaluation does not present a problem. However, 'because the very ambition of the goals, and the emphasis on holistic approaches arguably makes them vulnerable to attack, it is suggested that rigorous evaluation should not be avoided' (Harrison 1996: p9).

Table 4.1 *Selected Indicators for Evaluation of Healthy City Projects*

Driving force and pressure indicators

- Urban poverty level
- Crude birth and death rates
- Literacy levels, female and male
- Primary and secondary school enrolment rates
- Employment rate
- Average income levels and distribution
- Crime rate
- Atmospherics emissions (industry and traffic): heavy metals, gases, particulates
- Road traffic volumes, densities
- Untreated effluent
- Municipal, hazardous, medical waste products
- Amount of household waste not collected
- Number of illegal dump sites
- Electrification coverage
- Accidental release of toxic chemicals
- Indoor, outdoor air quality meet WHO standards
- Annual average visibility
- Water quality (drinking water quality standards met)
- Food quality (eg microbiological and chemical, pesticide residues)
- Heavy metals in air, water, solid, dust, food
- Crowding/living space
- Green spaces (surface area), distribution
- Community perceptions of environmental quality
- Noise levels

Exposure Indicators

Proportion of the population with:

- Safe drinking water (in home or 15 minutes walking distance)
- Access to regular garbage removal system
- Homes connected to a water supply system
- Substandard housing
- Overcrowded homes

Table 4.1 *Selected Indicators for Evaluation of Healthy City Projects (continued)*

- Informal (makeshift) housing
- No shelter (homeless)
- Homes connected to electricity supply
- Homes using biomass/coal for cooking/heating/lighting

Impact Indicators

- Crude death rate
- Infant mortality rate
- Neonatal, postnatal mortality
- Life expectancy at birth
- Cause specific death rates (eg deaths from diarrhoea, respiratory infection, asthma, traffic accidents, etc)
- Low birth weight babies
- Prevalence/incidence: respiratory-related diseases, diarrhoeal-related diseases, parasitic/infectious diseases, cardiovascular diseases, skin infections, mental ill health, work-related and traffic-related accidents

Process Indicators

- Existence of local environmental health policy and action plan
- Existence of local 'healthy public policies' which address environmental health issues
- Existence of Local Agenda 21 and other similar initiatives
- Existence of health/environmental policies in urban planning, housing, transport and other sectors
- Existence of emergency preparedness plans
- Existence of joint planning initiatives
- Urban renewal initiatives, settlement upgrading programmes
- Local standards/guidelines/legislation for food, air, water, hazardous substances, impact assessment, housing, etc.

Monitoring and Surveillance

- Existence of monitoring and surveillance systems for environmental (eg air, water) quality and food quality

Table 4.1 *Selected Indicators for Evaluation of Healthy City Projects (continued)*

- Existence of environmental health and health services information systems (with capacity for linkage)
- Capacity to track sentinel environmental diseases
- Capacity to track inequalities in environmental health status (age, gender, socio-economic status, etc)

Services Delivery

- Organization restructuring to integrate health and environment in decision making
- Environmental Health Officers (EHOs) per 10,000 population/district
- Proportion of environmental health personnel working in slum areas, informal sector, low income areas
- Proportion of population with access to environmental health services
- Decentralisation of decision-making structures
- Integrated service delivery mechanisms
- Immunization coverage rates
- Availability and accessibility of primary health care services
- Orientation towards preventive health services
- Emergency services
- Existence of supportive governmental structures at regional and national level

Budgeting and Finances

- Proportion of local city budget spent on health
- Proportion of local health budget spent on environmental health
- Sources of finances for environmental health
- Actions taken to mobilize additional resources for environmental health

Capacity Development

- City health education/health promotion programmes
- Food producers, handlers, sellers (including vendors) trained in basic food hygiene
- School education programmes in environmental health

Table 4.1 *Selected Indicators for Evaluation of Healthy City Projects (continued)*

- On-going environmental health/hygiene training programmes for EHOs, assistants, nurses, community health workers, engineers, planners, community groups in topics related to water and sanitation, waste disposal, vector control, food safety, chemical safety
- Career structures for environmental health personnel

Community Participation
- Mechanisms to involve stakeholders in decision making/policy development (eg formation of intersectoral steering committee)
- Joint planning initiatives (eg workshops, meetings held, stakeholder participation, etc)
- Women represented in planning and implementation of programmes and projects
- End-user participation in project formulation
- Communication networks for environmental health
- Existence of systems for dissemination of public information
- Inventories of environmental health organizations.

Source: Adapted from WHO (1996d)

Harrison then goes on to advocate various principles including the measurement of outcomes in terms of behavioural shifts (for example, lowering the smoking rate or increasing use of toilets and hygienic practices) where it is known that such shifts contribute to health gain (then no further demonstration of impact is needed); and a focus on the processes of inter-agency working and capacity building. Thus, he comes down in favour of process indicators.

In short, for the reasons noted above, evaluation of healthy city projects should be strongly based on process indicators which focus on the institutional and participatory aspects of the project (Werna and Harpham 1995). Impact indicators can be used on a complementary basis some years after implementation. The choice of the specific impact indicators will depend on the local circumstances as well as the timing of the evaluation (ie some indicators may measure change after say, two years (for example, mental health status), others will need nearer to five years (for example, infant mortality rate)). However, the problem of attributing change, as measured by impact indicators, to the intervention remains an issue (see Schrettenbrunner and Harpham 1993).

In order to define specific indicators to evaluate healthy city projects, it is also important to review a debate encountered in the healthy city literature: whether to use international indicators, or to generate them locally.

LOCAL VERSUS INTERNATIONAL INDICATORS

WHO publications recommend indicators (whether process or/and impact) which should be used in healthy city project evaluations throughout the world. These are here termed 'international indicators', and some are illustrated in Table 4.1.

However, the book edited by Davies and Kelly (1993), the major publication on healthy city project evaluation to date, criticizes the use of international indicators, and suggests that there is a need to develop local indicators for each specific project. It is argued that the local community should participate in the design of indicators as well as in the process of evaluation. Such a process would have value in itself, for involving the community. A recent WHO symposium (1997a) discussed the ownership of healthy city evaluations and the fact that it was important that cities' needs be taken into account as they are the ones who will have to make policy changes based on the evaluation results. Evaluation has a political dimension, ie it reflects power relations, which should be taken into account. It also entails conflict (between the actors involved). This should be brought to the surface rather than suppressed.

A further advantage of local indicators is that they counterbalance potential international biases. Evaluations in general and process indicators in particular are prone to value judgement. To give one example, criteria for assessing 'good performance of a given urban agency' designed by a Western researcher might differ from those established by local communities. Thus, the inclusion of the latter in the design of indicators (and in the evaluation process) is likely to balance the perspective taken.

Davies and Kelly's book (1993) also includes criticisms of inter-city evaluation, due to the specificity of each case. However, this is contentious. Inter-city comparisons are used widely, for instance in local government research. They might not provide an all-inclusive evaluation, but could be worth using in conjunction with other indicators. It is important to have some 'control method' for the evaluation. For example, a comparison over time or between places. A situation analysis at the outset would be a good solution and is covered in Chapter 3. However, when this is not possible, comparisons between different cities or towns where healthy city projects have been implemented could be used. However, it is important to stress that it is the comparison between cities that is useful and not a comparative evaluation. The latter is not appropriate given that projects are not in competition, that they have different starting points, that activities are not replicated and that much can be learnt (not copied) from other cities.

Inter-urban comparisons are important to detect problems (and possible solutions) and also to enable inter-city/town co-operation (which is a major issue in the healthy city movement). However, the sole use of local indicators in evaluations is likely to restrict such comparisons due to the specificity of the indicators. Thus, international indicators have an important role under such circumstances.

International indicators also have a further role when the local community is not prepared to design indicators and undertake evaluations. The authors who have written in favour of local indicators and community participation base their arguments on experiences from industrialized countries. However, many communities in developing countries are not prepared for such an involvement. It may take a long time for them to absorb the concept of healthy cities, let alone to participate in its evaluation. This has been noted, for instance in a preparatory assessment for the implementation of healthy city projects in developing countries, and in the first studies of individual projects in these countries (Werna and Harpham 1995).

The debate about local versus international indicators is partly about power and ownership of evaluations. This is considered further in the next section.

VALUES IN EVALUATION

The issue of values in evaluation is rarely discussed, let alone written about. However, Harrison (1996) points out that the issue of the ownership and control of the research agenda is one frequently discussed in relation to healthy city projects.

> 'This fertile debate has been stimulated by both the philosophical roots of the movement, by its engagement with communities and with action at a localised scale which inevitably brings into focus the links between values and evaluation and the deeper problems of the relationship between knowledge and power. The more general literature on policy evaluation also makes clear the potential for conflict over how and on what terms evaluation should be carried out between different interested parties and stakeholders' (Harisson 1996: p6).

Harrison then emphasizes that some critics of current evaluation methods argue that some sets of values do have privileged status, particularly when it comes to evaluating the worthiness of different projects for the spending of public funds. Rejections of cost benefit analyses and emphasis on attributing monetary values to policies are common. The New Economics Foundation, for example, suggests that current indicators which monitor sustainable development neglect to use indicators such as property rights, and participation in decision making and institutional capacity. Harrison (1996) says there is a need to accept into the evaluation arena a multiplicity of values and to accept that there will be difficult trade-offs to make in decision making. This thorny issue is yet to be encountered in developing countries, given the early stage of implementation of healthy city projects. However, it is necessary to bear these issues in mind when designing an evaluation.

DESIGNING AN EVALUATION – CONCLUSIONS

Evaluations of healthy city projects raise a multitude of issues. Harrison suggests that healthy city projects:

> 'represent "intervention" in social life and so beg questions of *effectiveness*, of what would have happened without such an intervention and whether they provide "additionality". They involve a commitment of resources and so raise issues of *efficiency* and whether those resources could have been better used. They involve *different interests* who will be concerned to see the evaluation process informed by different sets of *values* – consequently they raise *ethical* issues. Because the costs and benefits of such policies fall on different groups in different ways they raise issues of *equity*. They raise questions of to whom the evaluators are *accountable*. Questions of *methodology* relating, for example, to output as opposed to process based evaluation are posed. Also problems of which *criteria* to use and of what will be appropriate *indicators* will be confronted' (1996: p3).

This list of issues can be usefully used as a prompt in the design of an evaluation, to ensure that all key issues are addressed. Most of the issues have been addressed in this chapter. The costs of healthy city projects have never been examined and future evaluations should attempt costing exercises. Another point to bear in mind is that evaluation must be planned from the outset and not as an afterthought or when funding agencies request one.

The debate about healthy city project evaluations continues. In 1996 a meeting was held on 'Evaluating Healthy Cities Initiatives' in Bristol, UK. The debate at that meeting reflects the latest thinking and controversies with regards to evaluation in this field although it was limited to Europe. Agis Tsouros of the European office of the WHO explained that there were four elements to a healthy city project:

(1) endorsement of principles and strategies (for example Local Agenda 21);

(2) a commitment to local goals and changes (elaboration of a health profile, setting targets, developing a health plan, stimulating participation);
(3) establishment of project infrastructure (steering committee, co-ordination committees, focal points);
(4) networking (at the local, city, national and international levels).

Tsouros emphasized that it is at Point (2) where evaluation comes in although this excludes evaluating the wider influence of the project, for example on the ministry of health or country WHO office. He proposed (see also WHO 1997a) that the frame of reference for evaluation should be the health for All strategy, the 11 qualities of a healthy city (see Box 4.1), the designation requirements for the second phase of a healthy city, and the four action elements of the project (political commitment, visibility for health, institutional changes and innovative programmes). He then suggested that the elements of evaluation might be policy change, health profiles, plans, activities in health promotion and environmental health, networking, project management and organizational development.

Box 4.1 The Qualities of a Healthy City

A city should strive to provide:

1. A clean, safe physical environment of high quality (including housing quality).
2. An ecosystem that is stable now and sustainable in the long term.
3. A strong, mutually supportive and non-exploitative community.
4. A high degree of participation and control by the public over the decisions affecting their lives, health and well-being.
5. The meeting of basic needs (for food, water, shelter, in home, safety and work) for all the city's people.
6. Access to a wide variety of experiences and resources, with the chance for a wide variety of contact, interactions and communication.
7. A diverse, vital and innovative city economy.

> 8. The encouragement of connectedness with the past, with the cultural and biological heritage of city dwellers and with other groups and individuals.
> 9. A form that is compatible with and enhances the preceding characteristics.
> 10. An optimum level of appropriate public health and sick care services accessible to all.
> 11. High health status (high levels of positive health and low levels of disease).
>
> Source: WHO (1997a)

Tsouros emphasized some key considerations in evaluation which were the expectations of stakeholders, different interests within the city, the production of something useful to cities and the production of knowledge for the broader healthy city movement. It can be seen that many of these key considerations reflect the issues addressed in the current chapter. If an evaluation was constrained by limited resources, which is likely to be the case in developing countries, Tsouros suggested concentrating on three things:

(1) undertaking an annual peer review as opposed to an evaluation;
(2) enabling local research partner institutions to undertake some of the work; and
(3) seeking only evidence of policy shifts, changes in process, and examination of who the stakeholders are and how they have effected change.

The current chapter has discussed how to evaluate healthy city projects and has concluded by highlighting an alternative, minimalist approach. The present reality of developing countries may indeed require such minimalism due to the constraints in undertaking a more comprehensive approach. However, the advantages of comprehensive evaluation should not be forgotten and the feasibility of implementing such an evaluation should be regularly re-assessed.

5 Are Healthy Cities Sustainable?

The previous chapters presented what can be regarded as a full cycle of a healthy city project, starting with its organization, implementation, and finally evaluation. The last step, evaluation, feeds back, in order to re-initiate the cycle. Now, it is important to ask whether and how such a cycle could be re-initiated, and, ultimately, turned into a continuous process. In other words: are healthy cities sustainable?

This chapter addresses the above question, which has different dimensions (ie the environmental, economic, social dimensions of sustainability). It starts by reviewing the literature on sustainability in urban development and health, thus preparing the ground for the specific discussion about healthy city projects. The next section highlights characteristics of healthy cities which contribute to their sustainability. Subsequently, two case studies are presented in order to illustrate the discussion.

SUSTAINABILITY IN URBAN DEVELOPMENT AND HEALTH

The contemporary discussion about sustainable development in general started in the 1970s, focusing on the environmental impact of development policies (see, for example, Meadows et al 1974; Sachs 1979; Schumaker 1973; Ward and Dubos 1972, see also Mitlin 1992, for a review). There were loose or no references to urban issues within this general discussion (for example, Atkinson 1994; Hardoy et al 1992). However, the concept of sustainability eventually found its way into the specific literature on urban development.

The discussion about sustainable urban development also started with a strong environmental bias, for example, examining how cities and towns have affected the physical milieu through hazardous activities such as pollution and exhaustion of non-renewable resources. Issues regarding both the construction of urban areas (for instance, building materials, construction techniques, patterns of land occupation) and their maintenance (for example, supply of urban services, consumption habits) were explored in this way.

However, the discussion about sustainable development in general and about its specific application in the urban field eventually went beyond the environmental domain, thus encompassing economic, social, political and/or cultural aspects (see, for example, Atkinson 1994; Bhatti 1988; Brugman 1994; Hardoy et al 1992). Also, a multi-actor view has evolved, ie the belief that different actors such as local authorities, NGOs, community-based organizations (CBOs), etc play specific roles and have to be involved for the achievement of sustainable urban development.

Another important advancement in the sustainable urban development literature was the disaggregation of the two components of sustainable development, and the identification of an intrinsic conflict between the idea of sustaining something, which entails conservation, and the idea of developing it, which entails change. Hardoy et al (1992) provide a good clarification of this conflict. The term sustainable should be used mainly in reference to ecological sustainability, because:

'Sustaining societies or cultures is more ambiguous. Indeed, the achievement of many social, economic and political development goals requires fundamental changes to social structures including government institutions and, in many instances, to the distribution of assets and income' (Hardoy et al 1992: pp177–178).

Therefore, instead of applying the concept of sustainability to every single activity, one should note that 'what is important is that the sum (or net effect) of the activities within a specific area is sustainable' (Hardoy et al 1992: p182). Following, the sustainability of urban areas relates to their impact on environmental capital, and the developmental component relates to their performance and that of their institutions in catering for the needs of the population (such needs also include, but are not limited to, environmental issues such as protection from different types of pollution).

The literature has not reached a consensus regarding which specific issues should be sustainable and which issues should develop. However, the point to emphasize now is that the concept of sustainable urban development has been elaborated far beyond the environmental domain, including other fundamental aspects (political, cultural, etc) on their own and/or associated with environmental/ecological aspects, and also encompassing a multi-actor approach. As will be shown later, such a broad approach is important for the discussion about sustainable urban health in general and about the Healthy City Project in particular.

Despite the aforementioned elaborations regarding sustainable urban development, it is important to note that a significant number of authors and policy making agencies still have a strong environmental bias (see, for example, Choguill 1996; Leitman 1994; Serageldin and Cohen 1994; Stren et al 1992; UNCHS 1990; White 1994). This part of the sustainable urban development literature does refer to economy, politics, culture and society. However, it discusses such issues *within* an environmental/ecological perspective, for instance, the economic, political, cultural and/or social aspects of environmental sustainability. Of course this is not the same as discussing the sustainability and developmental aspects of these issues *on their own* and/or *associated with* environmental/ecological issues.

How does this discussion about sustainable urban development relate to sustainable urban health? In order to address this question, first the relationship between urban health and urban development needs to be clarified. The current concept of health is distant from (and much broader than) the traditional view which emerged in industrialized societies in the mid-20th century. The traditional view narrowly treats health care (which is an activity) as a synonym of health itself (which is a state of being), and places emphasis on the cure of diseases (for example, CCC–WHO 1993). The WHO epitomizes the current concept by defining health as a state of complete physical, social and mental well-being – which is much more than the mere absence of disease or infirmity; the attainment of which therefore requires far more than the supply of health services. Thus 'That health is a state of well-being indicates that health is not an activity ... rather it is the outcome of all activities which make up the lives of individuals, households, communities and cities' (CCC–WHO 1993: p3).

Such a statement, when applied to the specific realm of urban settlements, shows the importance of the different aspects of urban development to health. For instance:

'Physical, economic, social, and cultural aspects of city life all have an important influence on health. They exert their effect through such processes as population movement, industrialisation, and changes in the architectural and physical environment and in social organisation. Health is also affected in particular cities by climate, terrain, population density, housing stock, the nature of the economic activity, income distribution, transport systems, and opportunities for leisure and recreation' (WHO 1993: pp10–11).

In sum, it is necessary to act upon the several issues which constitute a city/town in order to improve the health of its citizens. Consequently, an approach to sustainable urban development which is able to connect such a wide range of issues may constitute a solid basis for achieving sustainable urban health and, by comparison, a unisectoral approach to sustainable urban development is bound to have notable constraints. Finally, it is worth mentioning that the causal relations between urban development and health also work the other way around. For instance, solutions to some major and specific health problems (for example, disease epidemics combated via improvements in water, sanitation, drainage and solid waste collection) can play an important role in a larger development strategy. For example, in Chittagong (a city which will be analysed later in this chapter) the improvements made in addressing these issues have supported the concomitant strategies of developing the city as a tourist destination, and also the rapid expansion of a number of industries. Therefore, there is a strong synergy between urban development and health.

As shown before, there have been different approaches to sustainable urban development, from a specific focus on environmental issues to a much wider focus. Paying attention to the environment is by all means fundamental. However, a specific concern with this aspect of sustainable urban development will exclude other issues which are also pivotal for addressing sustainable urban health, such as education, employment, domestic and street violence, recreation habits, to name a few.

THE SUSTAINABLE CHARACTERISTICS OF THE HEALTHY CITY PROJECT

Does the Healthy City Project address the issues discussed in the previous section?

There is a major debate within both the health and urban development fields which disputes the effectiveness of the denominated 'vertical' versus 'horizontal' approaches. This section argues that the Healthy City Project is more akin to the latter approach, which is likely to be more sustainable than the former. The traditional view of both health and urban development resulted in largely vertical interventions, which can be defined as having specific, usually quantifiable objectives related to a single condition or small group of health and/or urban problems; a focus on the short or medium term; and centralized management (see, for instance, Cairncross et al 1997, for a review of the health field). Examples of such interventions in the health field include eradication programmes of specific diseases such as poliomyelitis, neonatal tetanus, iodine and vitamin A deficiency, dracunculiasis or dengue. Examples in the urban development field include sectoral projects such as the construction of new estates to accommodate evicted slum dwellers, which focus only on the residential aspects of the 'slum problem'. Although there have been some successes associated with vertical interventions, in general their objectives have been limited in scope and, relative to the resources used, there have been few long-term gains for low income population groups. As Cairncross et al (1997) suggest in their analysis of the health field, vertical programmes suit donor requirements in some ways, such as ease of evaluation, and there are circumstances where they may be advantageous, such as eradication campaigns where results can be achieved quickly, and disease control activities requiring complex or expensive technology. However, the aforementioned authors argue that there should be no assumption that vertical programmes offer sustainable benefits besides their primary objectives, and the case that they allow greater efficacy in the supply of disease control measures is not proven. A similar argument could be developed for vertical programmes in the urban development field.

The Healthy City Project framework is more akin to interventions derived from the denominated horizontal approach, such as encouraging community participation, working across sectors, local capacity building, making links between the environment and health. Examples of horizontal interventions include integrated slum improvement programmes, community development programmes, overall health sector reforms such as the Bamako Initiative, overall municipal administration reforms, among others. Such horizontal interventions may be more difficult to evaluate than vertical ones (see Chapter 4) and may need longer time spans to produce results. Yet, they often induce systemic changes, which are in line with the concepts of sustainability discussed in the previous section.

The point here is not to dismiss totally the possible advantages of the vertical approach, which have been mentioned before, but to concentrate on its sustainability aspects. It is also interesting to note that in a number of instances, vertical and horizontal approaches could be integrated, such as the case of health workers (horizontal) acting under the co-ordinated supervision of, and support from, the health centre and district levels (vertical) (Cairncross et al 1997). This is an interesting issue to be pursued through further investigation, as its elaboration falls beyond the scope of this book.

In short, this chapter argues that the horizontal approach is more likely to be sustainable. However, it will not try to demonstrate such a statement through empirical evidence or otherwise. This would require a different type of research. Rather, the chapter puts forward such a statement as an assumption, which was generated through the conceptual reasoning developed in the text. The chapter will in fact demonstrate that – and how – the Healthy City Project includes a number of aspects, which, according to the argument developed here, are central to achieving sustainability.

The WHO (1995a) has identified two key aspects that help define the Healthy City Project: intersectoral collaboration for health, and supportive environments. In terms of intersectoral collaboration, agencies concerned with energy, food, economic planning, housing, land use, transportation and other areas are required to examine the health implications of their policies and programmes, and adjust them to better promote health and a healthy environment. The WHO acknowledges that such collaboration has failed a number of times because it was unclear how the health sector was to be involved, and there was little political support. It is suggested (WHO 1995a) that such collaboration requires (1) a measurement of the health impacts of various development activities; (2) policies on health for particular settings (housing, workplaces, schools, etc); and (3) advocacy by the health sector in relation to each implementing ministry or agency. The more successful healthy city projects have obtained political support by involving mayors, universities, NGOs, private companies and community organizations. This partnership then contributes to the formation of a City Health Plan (presented in chapters 1 and 2).

The idea of a supportive environment and the settings approach (see Chapter 1), in turn, is based on the premise that health status is determined more by conditions in certain settings such as work, school, home than by the health care services or facilities that are provided. There is now an increasing use of settings based on 'multi-city action plans', for issues such as school health or food market health, whereby cities in a network exchange experiences and information materials about addressing specific issues. WHO regional offices are increasingly involved in such networking activities.

The above description of the healthy city concept emphasizes a number of characteristics that can contribute to sustainable urban health, namely a broad definition of health, an intersectoral approach and the involvement of a wide range of actors. These issues are in line with the horizontal approach previously discussed. An additional important characteristic is that the WHO provides limited external funding and instead places emphasis on mobilizing local resources.

The emphasis of many international programmes on large provisions of external funds has in many instances created an image that international assistance is necessarily a synonym for money. Following, many local authorities in developing countries have adapted their behaviour to such a situation, in the sense that they welcome external funds in their cities, but do not necessarily welcome other types of assistance (such as technical training) nor are they willing to mobilize local resources. However, a large number of external funds-oriented programmes have encountered serious problems (for example, Harris 1992; Werna 1996c). This is because a major focus on external financial resources has often overshadowed the need to build local capacity to manage such resources and indeed to continue activities after the end of the international project, therefore re-fuelling the need for more external money and re-strengthening the aforementioned type of behaviour among local authorities. Under these circumstances, an emphasis on the mobilization of local resources may bring a systemic change which will capacitate local stakeholders not only to depend less on external support, but also to manage their own resources better. It also broadens the approach to sustainability, often used by donor agencies, which merely focuses on the ability of government authorities of a developing country to continue activities after the withdrawal of funding from multilateral or bilateral agencies. The idea of mobilizing local resources is a fundamental component of the Healthy

City Project, and is in line with the horizontal approach, see, for instance, the comparison between levels of external funds used in vertical as opposed to horizontal interventions in Cairncross et al (1997).

In short, four sustainability characteristics have been identified throughout this section. Evidence of their presence in the Healthy Cities Project will be presented in the next section, through the analysis of two case studies, Chittagong and Bangkok.

CASE STUDY: CHITTAGONG, BANGLADESH

The main features of Chittagong and its Healthy City Project have already been presented in Chapter 2. The attributes of this Project in respect to sustainable urban health are explained below.

A Broad Definition of Health

A broad definition of health, as already noted, is a basic tenet of the Healthy City Project concept itself. The very fact that the Chittagong Healthy City Project includes a wide range of actors (most of whom are not linked to health services) and intersectoral activities (explained below) confirms the adoption of such a broad approach.

Experiences in developing countries have shown that such a broad approach is not easily understood by the actors responsible for the several aspects of urban development, and by the population in general. Equating the Healthy City Project solely with improvements in health services – as opposed to overall urban improvements – is the most common (although not the only) problem. Thus, the broad concept of health has been widely explained in Chittagong, through; (1) seminars and workshops with the participation of professionals with expertise in the Healthy City Project; (2) approaching the media; (3) the activities of local consultants; and (4) a wide distribution of key texts such as the Plan of Action of the Chittagong Healthy City Project (CCC–WHO 1993) and of newsletters (prepared by the local consultants). The importance of each specific aspect of the development of the city (housing, education, transport, culture, etc) to the health of the population has been emphasized through the methods mentioned above, so that the actors responsible for each one of them clearly understand their role (and those of others) in the process.

The adoption of a broad definition of health also means that the local co-ordinator of a healthy city project does not have to be a medical doctor, or any other professional linked to health services. A primary requisite for a co-ordinator, in addition to leadership skills, is a deep understanding of the process of urban development and of its impact on the well-being of the citizens – rather than expertise in health/medical services. As noted in Chapter 2, in Chittagong the initial co-ordinator was a magistrate of the City Corporation, who was succeeded by a civil engineer belonging to the same local authority. Such a choice of co-ordinators substantiates the adoption of a broad definition of health in the Chittagong Healthy City Project. At the same time, it helps to clarify to the lay public that the Healthy City project is not specifically related to health services.

Intersectoral Activities

This element is illustrated by the type, range of, and integration between, topics and actions which constitute the Chittagong Healthy City Project. First, as noted in Chapter 2, this Project is formed by seven sectoral task forces, which encompass the major fields of urban development in Chittagong.

Also, improvements in the aforementioned areas are to be achieved by the implementation of a multisectoral Plan of Action comprising 73 specific activities as diverse as a transport development strategy, a mechanism to attract inward investment to Chittagong, community business investment support mechanisms, extension of technical and vocational training, legislation to prevent hill cutting, support for rag pickers to sell and distribute low cost latrines, to name a few (CCC–WHO 1993). The comprehensiveness of these activities as well as their interrelationship are explicit in the Plan of Action, which states that if any parts of this package are missing, the overall effectiveness of the Chittagong Healthy City Project may be compromised (CCC–WHO 1993).

Wide Range of Actors

The institutional organization of the Chittagong Project reflects the involvement of a wide range of actors. As noted in Chapter 2, in addition to an office (headed by the co-ordinator), the Project includes a steering committee and task forces.

The steering committee is formed by the main organizations from all sectors (ie the public, community, voluntary and private sectors as well as international agencies, see Box 2.1) which are involved in the different aspects of the development of Chittagong. Bottom-up participation is particularly encouraged (CCC–WHO 1993).

Each sectoral task force is constituted by all the actors involved in the specific field. For instance, the Water and Sanitation Task Force is formed by the Chittagong Water Development Authority, the Department of Engineering of the City Corporation, all the NGOs and CBOs with activities in this field, among others.

The Chittagong Healthy City Project also includes zonal task forces, responsible for the plans and actions in specific geographical areas of the city. They are constituted by all the social actors with a strong concern with each area, for example, local councillors, all NGOs and CBOs with projects in the area, informal/traditional community leaders. There is indeed overlap between actors in sectoral and zonal task forces. However, this does not constitute a problem. By integrating the plans of the sectoral task forces with those of the zonal task forces, the overall Plan of Action of the Healthy City Project is formulated.

The actors involved in the Chittagong Project are outlined in Table 5.1. The Plan of Action (CCC–WHO 1993) includes details of the roles of each of these actors.

Limited External Funding

Funding given by the WHO to the Chittagong Healthy City Project has been restricted to setting up the office (for example, furniture and equipment), technical advice (for example, local consultants and short-term international consultants to assist in capacity building) and field studies commissioned to local academics.

The fact that the Healthy City Project is not about bringing 'a basket full of money' to Chittagong has been emphasized since the inception of the Project in this city. This has led local actors to take more sustainable routes. In 1994 the City Corporation initiated a number of activities in a pilot area (which it termed Healthy Ward) with its own resources. Also, a number of development projects (for example, eight maternal and childcare centres)

Are Healthy Cities Sustainable?

Table 5.1 *Actors Involved in the Chittagong Health City Project*

Public sector	Private sector	NGOs	Community organizations	Internatl orgs
Bakrabad Gas Co Technology	Chamber of Commerce	ADAB	Community associations	UNCHS
Bangladesh Railway	Leading banks	Concern NGO Forum	Slum leaders	UNDP
Bangladesh Road Transport Corporation	Lions Club Rotary Club	World Vision Other NGOs to be incorporated later on		UNICEF WHO
Chittagong City Corporation				
Chittagong Development Authority				
Chittagong University				
Civil Surgeon				
Defence Service				
Department of Environment				
Department of Forests				
Export Processing Zone				
Facilities Department				
Housing and Settlement Directorate				
Liquidified Petroleum Gas Plant				
Ministry of Health				
Port Authority				
Power Development Board				
Primary/Secondary/ Higher Education Depts				
Public Works Department				
Roads and Highways Department				

Source: CCC–WHO (1993)

to be considered for external funding have been under discussion by the Chittagong Project partners. It has been a *sine qua non* condition that the identification of such development activities and the initiative to seek external funding should be taken by the local actors, and not spoonfed top-down by the WHO.

CASE STUDY: BANGKOK, THAILAND

The Bangkok Metropolitan Administration (BMA 1994) has identified the priority urban health problems as environmental pollution, solid waste management and malnutrition. In 1994 the BMA identified three districts within Bangkok in which to start a healthy city project. Two key objectives were to mobilize participation and networks between government and private sectors and to improve health through enhanced living conditions in key settings (namely housing, workplace, schools and food outlets). A key outcome identified by the BMA is the formulation of a sustainable process of urban development that enhances cultural heritage (BMA 1994).

A Broad Definition of Health

In its background to the Bangkok Healthy City Project, the BMA has explicitly stated the recognition of the interaction between physical, mental, social and spiritual dimensions of health. One of the desired outcomes is that community members can co-operatively identify existing resources to enable them to support each other mutually in improving their quality of life in relation to infrastructure, socio-economic status, physical health status, mental health and environmental well-being.

Intersectoral Activities

The nature of the intersectoral action being undertaken in the Bangkok Healthy City Project can be illustrated by one of its activities: that of the 'healthy and safe workplace' programme. This operates at two levels: one, the traditional occupational health service that emphasizes factory-level work by health inspectors; and two, the newer challenge of the small-scale and cottage industries that are not amenable to traditional approaches and that demand community-based and participatory approaches that may best be implemented by local government with national government support (BMA 1994). Goldstein (in BMA 1994) identifies issues that such a programme will address (see Chapter 3).

To meet such objectives alone, a variety of sectors have been involved and this takes the Healthy City Project outside the ministry of health or the BMA's health department. It should be noted that metropolitan authorities are often in a stronger position to undertake multisectoral action given

Are Healthy Cities Sustainable?

the variety of departments under their mandate. Activities and projects within the ministry of health often suffer because such ministries may be isolated and weak in relation to other ministries at the central government level (see also the discussion about the role of the health sector in Chapter 2).

Wide Range of Actors

Figure 5.1 demonstrates the actors in the Bangkok Healthy City Project. The inner circle represents the Project's committee, while the middle ring represents the various departments of the BMA which are brought together for the Project. The outer ring represents other organizations and actors contributing to the Project within Bangkok. This demonstrates the wide range of actors involved.

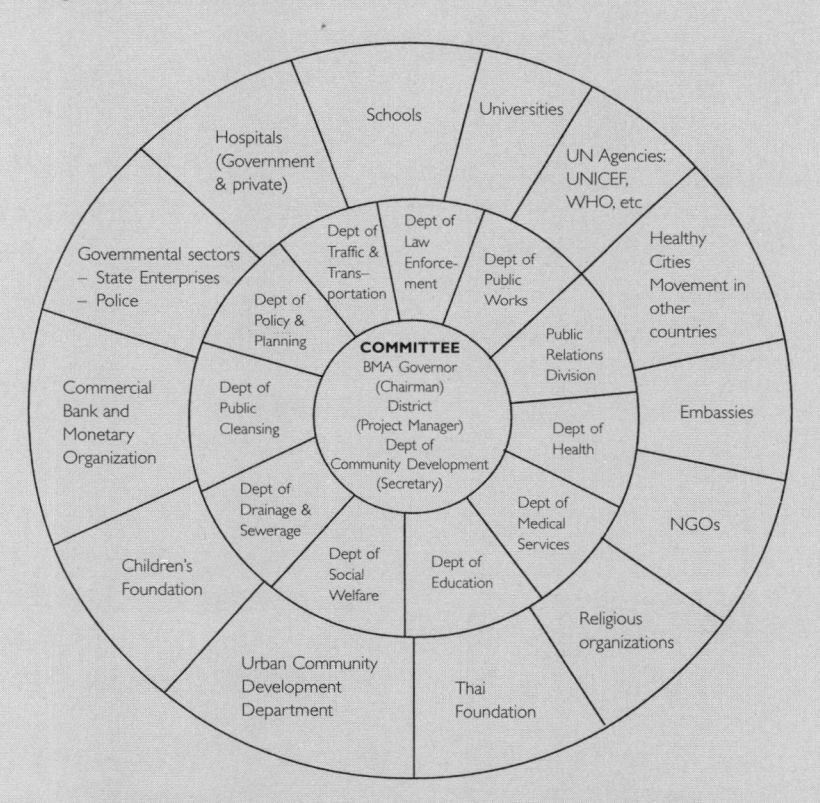

Figure 5.1 *The Actors in Bangkok Healthy City Project.*

Source: Harpham and Werna (1996a)

Limited External Funding

Similarly to Chittagong, Bangkok has relied mostly on local resources. In 1994 a budget of nearly 4 million baht (approximately US$160,000) was approved. It aimed at covering the 20 steps for developing a healthy city project, given in Figure 5.2. Additional (international) funding is currently being obtained by a local university to undertake a costing exercise of the Bangkok Project. Such an exercise addresses a criticism that has been levelled at the healthy city initiative, ie that there is no evidence of what the initiative costs in real terms (for example participation of various actors involved).

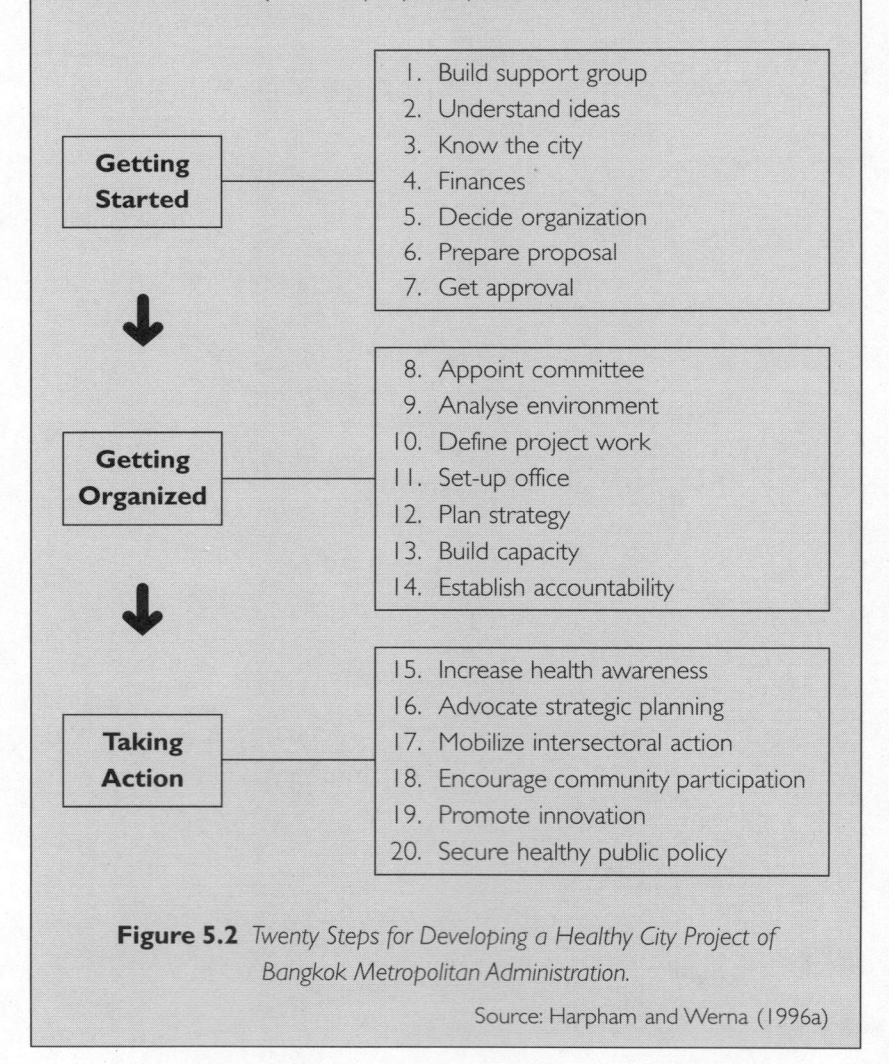

Getting Started
1. Build support group
2. Understand ideas
3. Know the city
4. Finances
5. Decide organization
6. Prepare proposal
7. Get approval

Getting Organized
8. Appoint committee
9. Analyse environment
10. Define project work
11. Set-up office
12. Plan strategy
13. Build capacity
14. Establish accountability

Taking Action
15. Increase health awareness
16. Advocate strategic planning
17. Mobilize intersectoral action
18. Encourage community participation
19. Promote innovation
20. Secure healthy public policy

Figure 5.2 *Twenty Steps for Developing a Healthy City Project of Bangkok Metropolitan Administration.*

Source: Harpham and Werna (1996a)

CONCLUSION

This chapter has analysed sustainability in urban development and health, and the Healthy City Project was presented as a significant initiative in this respect. Four attributes of the healthy city project have been particularly noted. However, the emphasis on a broad definition of health, intersectoral activities, a wide range of actors and limited funding does not embody a claim that all possible factors required for sustainability have been identified here. As a suggestion for the improvement of the Healthy City Project, this chapter will end with an analysis of the supra-local dimension of urban sustainability.

The literature on sustainable urban development shows that it is important to have a broad approach not only in an intra-urban sense. It is also vital to have an approach on a multi-layer/supra-urban sense, because cities and towns are dependent upon and influenced by regional, national and international factors such as macroeconomic policies, recession, capital flows, trade, technology transfer, to name a few (for example, Atkinson 1994; Hardoy et al 1992; White 1994). The importance of the impact of supra-urban issues on the specific realm of urban health has been noted as well (for example, Werna et al 1996).

Thus, only part of the actions to achieve sustainable urban development and health lies within the control of cities and towns themselves (and the Healthy City Project has been comprehensive regarding this set of actions). However, another important part lies outside the local realm: changes in the supra-urban issues which affect urban areas, and also the particular roles for supra-urban actors to boost changes within cities or towns.

It is suggested here that the Healthy City Project will be further strengthened by giving more attention to the supra-urban issues. Of course the supra-urban activities of healthy city projects have limits. However, there are more feasible actions that could be taken. For instance, actions in the realm of supra-urban national authorities which affect the places where the Project is being implemented. To give one example, as noted in Chapter 2, in Chittagong there are many public agencies connected to eight different ministries, which are involved in several aspects of the administration of the city and in the provision of its public services. These agencies are not accountable to the City Corporation, which co-ordinates the Chittagong Healthy City Project. Intersectoral action within Chittagong does ameliorate this problem. However, there is still a need for action to be taken in Dhaka, the capital city of Bangladesh, ie action at the ministries' level (see Werna 1995a).

Other papers on the subject of sustainability (Harpham and Werna 1996a, 1996b) have highlighted that supra-urban actions can be carried out via two complementary methods: (1) the involvement of the supra-urban actors (for example, federal and regional governments); and (2) the activities of local actors outside the urban/local domain. The first method has had much more attention in the literature. However, despite its relative neglect, the second method is also important. The two aforementioned papers have shown the need for local actors to 'think locally and act globally': to take the local issues that they know well to broader forums and domains where consequential decisions are made. Healthy city projects themselves, through their burgeoning networks, may be a strong lever for local actors to implement wider actions.

Networking among healthy city projects in developing countries is already a reality, and should be strengthened further. As communications improve, there are now examples of healthy city projects where co-ordinators are able to receive information about urban issues and successful experiences in cities from other regions by different means, even by e-mail or the Internet (for example, Dar es Salaam and Chittagong). Also, many co-ordinators are now attending international meetings on urban health with increasing frequency. This can have a desirable effect in encouraging local city projects to adopt policies and programmes that are strongly endorsed and promoted at international urban forums, such as participatory urban governance. Networking has the impact of creating a sense of belonging to a larger group or structure, and often seems to encourage involved individuals to make an extra effort to ensure their local project activities are effective. Thus the positive international

Are Healthy Cities Sustainable?

response to various innovations in Chittagong (such as the application of the pedalled three-wheeler solid waste vehicles, as reported in the 1997 Baltimore International Urban Health Conference) has stimulated the local staff to renew their efforts in many aspects of the programme. The role of networking may be of particular importance in those countries where the culture of local government service emphasizes hierarchical workgroups and lack of participation by lower level offices in decision making (let alone participation of outside bodies or NGOs in the process). Without the stimulus of networking that provides an influential support for participatory approaches, the implementation of healthy city projects and especially the parts such as coalitions around housing and health, school health, etc, may not be workable.

6 Conclusion

This book aimed to analyse the current state of healthy city projects in developing countries, and to make recommendations for the future. These aims have been met through a set of chapters which started with a historical and conceptual account of the Healthy City Project (the introductory chapter), followed by the analysis of its full cycle (the establishing, implementation and evaluation chapters), and finally the transformation of the cycle into a continuous process (the sustainability chapter). The current chapter will put together the main points presented throughout the book. These conclusions will be organized into five sections. These sections do not follow the same structure as the set of chapters, but cut across the main themes and reflect the recommendations put forward. The sections will make reference to the previous chapters, in order to help the reader understand the web of arguments that has been constructed. Although there is some overlap between the sections presented below, they do have specificities, and will be presented separately.

The first section focuses on the healthy city approach. The second, third and fourth sections focus on three main dimensions embodied in the Healthy City Project, namely: (1) an international initiative; (2) public administration; and (3) popular participation. To conclude, the fifth section discusses whether the Healthy City Project needs to exist indefinitely and what are the implications for the development of *healthy cities* beyond the *Project*.

Conclusion

THE HEALTHY CITY APPROACH

Chapter 1 investigated the sources of inspiration of the healthy city approach (for example, the sanitary ideology, Alma Ata, the Ottawa Charter, the Rio Summit). Integration or intersectoral action constitute a major thrust of such initiatives, and are a main pillar of healthy city projects, as noted in the same chapter. This section highlights problems related to the integrated or intersectoral approach, and makes related recommendations.

Although integration or intersectoral action are now widespread concepts both in urban development and in health, there are still significant difficulties in realizing them. Despite the fact that such concepts are by no means new, the WHO recently held a scientific meeting specifically to discuss how to implement intersectoral action in health. This convention highlighted the existence of many constraints, from the local to the global level (WHO 1996e, 1997b). The literature on urban development, in its turn, has focused on integration as perhaps *the* paradigm for the 1990s, as opposed to the previous focus on the project approach, which consists of scattered interventions implemented independently (for example, Harris, 1992; World Bank 1991; see Werna 1996c, for a review). However, documentation of sound implementation of integrated programmes of urban development is still rare.

A major difficulty in implementing integrated/intersectoral programmes, which is particularly prominent in developing countries, is the resistance of public authorities to move away from traditional sectoral/vertical ways of functioning (see Chapters 2 and 5). This is mainly connected with: (1) lack of knowledge about intersectoral action; and/or (2) line departments fearing interference from their counterparts in internal affairs.

The above situation may also take place, or be exacerbated, when integrated/intersectoral programmes are poorly conceptualized and designed. In this respect, it is worth noting that the discussion on integration or intersectoral action in the urban development literature is still vague. As mentioned before, the argument in favour of such an approach came about as a reaction to the project approach, which has had an unimpressive track-record of achievements despite many decades of implementation (for example, Harris 1992; Werna 1996c). There has been an emphasis on the problems associated with the implementation of such independent interventions, for example, overlaps, gaps and even conflicts between the activities of different line departments, and, perhaps most importantly, the fact that many urban problems are comprehensive in nature and cannot be addressed through dispersed actions. This situation, the argument goes, calls for integration of actions. However, perhaps because there has been a need for a strong reaction and counterpoint against fragmentation of urban actions, the integrated/intersectoral approach has overemphasized the holistic motto that in cities 'everything is related to everything else'. While such an argument is true in principle, the design of an integrated programme for a given city still requires disaggregation in order to address soundly its different aspects. Such a holistic idea, if taken to extremes, may confuse the design of programmes and may affect, for instance, the establishment of specific actions and priorities. A programme designer could be lead to think that it does not matter where and how to start, because everything is in the end related. On the other hand, s/he could overestimate the impact of a specific action, based on the thought that such an action is connected to everything else. The above reasoning is based not only on rational deduction but on casual observation and informal interviews with urban policy makers in developing countries.

An overemphasis on the holistic motto makes it hard for a given integrated programme to have a distinct personality: it is difficult to pinpoint the characteristics which distinguish a programme from others, as all of them address the same set of issues via the same basic approach.

Sound implementation of the integrated/intersectoral approach in urban development and health is still incipient, despite all the rhetoric. Therefore, the Healthy City Project should not be seen as yet another initiative which just uses such an approach. Rather, the Healthy City Projects can be regarded as a pioneer of the approach.

Conclusion

How can Healthy City projects address the problems associated with the (ill) design of an integrated/intersectoral programme? One solution is to organize the Project in each city or town around health issues which are perceived as important, and then build all the urban interlinkages around such a focus. This would avoid the vagueness that can arise from the view that everything is related to health and health is related to everything. It would therefore not matter how a project is designed. It is common to find mayors and their staff having difficulty in thinking beyond the holistic motto. Therefore, it is important for each healthy city project to have a clear focus from the beginning. The issues to be focused on vary from city to city, and should be chosen in a participatory manner – when the people involved have a vital stake in the issues being addressed, the initiatives are more likely to work.

As noted in Chapter 2, a major point of distinction between cities in developing and industrialized countries is that the former have fewer resources to deal with a larger set of problems thus emphasizing the need to choose priorities (Chapters 2 and 3). However, the implementation of priorities has to be carried out via specific projects. Therefore, are there differences between such projects and other projects which are traditionally found in any given city or town, outside the umbrella of Healthy Cities? One characteristic of healthy city projects is that they attend to the priorities of the population, following the principles of the City Health Plan (chapters 1, 2 and 3). This is not necessarily the case regarding other traditional projects, which may give priority to the interests of specific stakeholders. Another characteristic of healthy city projects is that they are not isolated or fragmented, but part of a network of ideas and related actions, which are expressed through the City Health Plan. Also, being participatory they enjoy broad support. Finally, they may also benefit from experiences in other healthy city projects through network contacts.

The concern with specific projects counteracting the integrated approach is reinforced by the use of settings in healthy cities (Chapter 3). As noted before, many healthy city projects have chosen to concentrate their actions on promoting specific healthy settings, such as schools, workplaces, market places, etc. Such actions, however, should not be designed in isolation, but as integral parts of the City Health Plan.

This section has considered the main thrust of the healthy city approach. It is now important to see how the Project has been realized in practice. Three main dimensions of this practice will be discussed in turn.

HEALTHY CITY PROJECTS AS AN INTERNATIONAL INITIATIVE

This dimension represents a main difference between the Healthy City Project in industrialized and developing countries. In the former set of countries, the involvement of the WHO can be less, due to the advanced (at least in relative terms) ability of the local stakeholders to assimilate the Project. Also, as noted in Chapter 2, and in the above section, these countries have larger resources to implement the Project. The WHO faces a different challenge in developing countries, where cities have few resources to address a large range of problems. This condition does not mean that the WHO has to bring in all the extra resources necessary to address all urban health problems of developing countries. But it does mean that in such countries the WHO faces different problems from the conditions found in the industrialized world and thus must operate differently. The Project has to be adapted because, as noted in Chapter 1, it originated in industrialized countries.

In addition to the aforementioned differences, in developing countries the Healthy City Project is encompassed within the international aid machinery. This fact represents a fundamental distinction vis-à-vis the situation in industrialized countries, because it entails a specific kind of relationship between the Project and the recipient cities. After a number of decades of international aid, a culture of aid has been established throughout the developing world. This has prompted the rise of a specific kind of behaviour within the public sector (and eventually the population in general) vis-à-vis international agencies. This behaviour sometimes creates problems, such as public authorities expecting paternalistic support from international agencies, or such agencies being suspected of interfering in internal affairs. No matter how Healthy City Projects may in reality differ from other/traditional international projects, local stakeholders and partners in developing countries are often not able to make the distinctions from the start. This situation must be taken into account, for the sound implementation of Healthy City Projects. The remainder of this section will analyse two further issues related to the international nature of the Healthy City Project and its presence in developing countries, ie (1) how to start a participatory process top-down; and (2) the place of the Healthy City Project among other international initiatives.

A recent encounter between a Mexican local politician and one of the authors of this book illustrates the first issue mentioned above. Despite the fact that Mexico has a very large number of healthy city projects (probably the largest in the developing world) and an active network, the politician criticized the Project for being conceptually – and in practice – contradictory, because, on the one hand, it claims popular participation; but, on the other hand, is a top-down international programme. In his opinion, these two sides are conflicting. This reflects a criticism that has often been made. Such criticism is not only levelled at the Healthy City Project, but numerous international initiatives which have a participatory ethos. This book argues against such criticism. First, there is a difference between top-down imposition of ideas, and facilitation of local initiatives. The healthy city project aims at the latter, not the former. Also, this book argues that in many circumstances a good idea or concept can successfully be transferred from one settlement to another. Otherwise, we would still be living in a world of isolated communities which would constantly be reinventing the wheel. The Healthy City Project has such a transfer of knowledge component which does not necessarily clash with local participation. One should still not let outside ideas constrain local initiatives. In other words, as mentioned in Chapter 2, the Healthy City Project needs to keep a balance between prescribing action for the cities/towns, and starving them of inputs.

Another issue related to the international nature of the Healthy City Project is its place among other international initiatives. There are many international initiatives which have an integrated/intersectoral approach. Examples include (UNCHS–UNEP 1996):

- Sustainable Cities Programme (run by UNCHS;
- Sustainable Cities Initiative (run by USAID, the United States Agency for International Development);
- Metropolitan Environmental Improvement Programme (run by the World Bank);
- International Center for Sustainable Cities (run by an NGO with the same name);
- CITYNET (run by the Regional Network of Local Authorities for the Management of Human Settlements);
- Private Public Partnership for the Urban Environment Programme (run by UNDP, in association with the Sustainable Project Management Programme and the Massachusetts Institute of Technology);
- Local Agenda 21 Initiative (run by ICLEI, the International Council for Local Environmental Initiatives).

The existence of multiple initiatives is not necessarily a problem. However, it needs good co-ordination (Werna 1996c), particularly when two or more programmes are concomitantly implemented in the same city, which has happened already, in Dakar, Senegal; Johannesburg, South Africa; Madras, India; among others (for example, UNCHS–UNEP 1997). Such a situation reinforces the need for the Healthy City Project to strengthen its character based on a clear focus on health issues. The Healthy City Project also needs to be flexible enough to be able to adapt itself to other integrated international programmes. The concomitant implementation of the Healthy City Project and the Sustainable City Programme in Ibadan (Nigeria) and the synergies created between them constitute a successful experience.

Conclusion

The previous section highlighted how the intersectoral approach is still problematic in many respects. It also highlighted how the Healthy City Project may address such problems. Therefore, other international programmes may learn useful lessons from the experiences of healthy cities. Such lessons may be related not only to issues of implementation, as already discussed, but also evaluation (Chapter 4), as the evaluation of integrated programmes is still a limited field of knowledge (see chapters 4 and 5).

HEALTHY CITY PROJECTS AS PUBLIC ADMINISTRATION

Although an international initiative, the Healthy City Project is not just owned by an international agency and applied in a given country. Rather, it is a programme in partnership with local stakeholders, with a major objective of promoting good health and preventing health-related problems at the local level via a systemic change in urban policies. Such an emphasis in change in policy entails the involvement of, and often transformations within, the public sector (Chapter 2). The local government is the leading agency/stakeholder in a healthy city project (Chapter 2). Therefore, public administration is an important dimension of Healthy Cities.

Experience shows that the internal dynamics of the public sector are a major determinant of success in a healthy city project in developing countries. In this regard, two major issues should be highlighted: (1) motivation of the public authorities; and (2) motivation of the staff of public agencies.

First, the political backing of local decision makers – especially mayors or their counterparts – is a key element in the implementation of healthy city projects. Conversely, a number of on-going projects have lost momentum precisely because of changes in the leadership of the local government, particularly when a given mayor is succeeded by a political opponent. Unfortunately, the dismantling of established and on-going programmes by an arriving government is a common practice in many countries. For instance, the Campinas Healthy City Project (noted in Chapter 3) has faced such a problem.

Healthy city projects facing the above problem can be supported by initiatives from outside the public administration system. Active popular participation is probably the best option, as the following section will argue. The WHO may also play an important role as, for example, it did in Chittagong (noted in chapters 2 and 5) – the Project in this city started in 1993, but one year later there was a radical political shift in the local government.

One possible solution with a focus on the public administration system entails an awareness raising campaign targeting new politicians, especially forthcoming mayors. The PAHO (Pan-American Health Organization) is currently discussing such an idea.

A second issue related to the internal dynamics of the public sector is the motivation of public employees. Staff of local government and other public agencies with a stake in urban affairs are often strongly involved in the day-to-day running and decision making of a healthy city project, for example, leading task forces, implementing activities of the City Health Plan (Chapter 2). Therefore, if not well motivated, such staff may jeopardize the implementation of a project. For example, there have been cases of public employees who had difficulty in incorporating the activities of the Healthy City Project into their routine duties. When this happens, Healthy City Projects can be regarded as an extra-assignment, a fact which disheartens the responsible public employees. Also, as noted in Chapter 2, successful projects in developing countries often entail changes in ways of working. This requires further motivation. A clear design of a healthy city project backed by steady political support and an awareness raising campaign targeting public staff may address this issue.

Taking into consideration that public administration is a fundamental dimension of Healthy City Projects, a vital question to ask is who will be the main partner of the WHO in the leadership of the Project in the future. In other words, which public entity in each country and city would be responsible. There are two major candidates: (1) the health sector; and (2) the local authorities.

The health sector has a major advantage of being the traditional partner of the WHO (ie via the national ministries of health). Also, there is of course a rationale for involving the health sector in a movement/programme which deals with promoting good health and preventing health-related problems (Chapter 2). However, the health sector also has a significant disadvantage. Healthy city projects entail policy making in many fields which are outside the control of public health authorities, such as housing, transport, education and employment.

Local authorities, in their turn, have the advantage of being responsible for urban policies in general, a fact which would enable them to act more effectively against the root causes of a plethora of health problems. They are also represented internationally, through the IULA (International Union of Local Authorities), which means that their support for healthy city projects can go beyond the local and national domain. But local authorities also have disadvantages, such as the lack of a traditional linkage with health as an issue and with the WHO as an organization. Their possible involvement in the Healthy City Project as a leading partner may also generate conflict with the public health sector (for example, with ministries of health) which would not want to lose their position as traditional partners of the WHO (also bearing in mind that the secretary-general of the WHO is chosen by the ministers of health).

In sum, there is no clear-cut picture about whether the health sector or local authorities should take the lead. Therefore, this book highlights the need for an action-space to discuss a possible solution. Chapter 2 alluded to a possible method to come to such a solution, ie rather than establishing beforehand who should lead the healthy city movement; it would be more appropriate to monitor the implementation of on-going healthy city projects around the world and identify the natural leaders that emerge from the movement.

HEALTHY CITY PROJECTS AS POPULAR PARTICIPATION

Although healthy city projects may be an international initiative as well as a means to conduct public administration, as noted in the previous sections, it is fundamentally about participatory governance. Chapter 5 concentrated on four issues related to the sustainability of healthy cities; a broad range of actors being one of them. Within this issue, popular participation may be the ultimate element which leads to, and supports, sustainability.

The preceding section noted that the success or failure of healthy city projects in developing countries has been largely associated with the degree of political support from local decision makers. In most cases, such support still does not fully reflect ideas coming from different sectors of the population. Grass roots initiatives exist, but many healthy city projects are still heavily linked to the personal agendas of mayors who have implemented them in the first place. Although the WHO and indeed many mayors have taken popular participation as a fundamental element of healthy city projects, in reality its implementation is frequently not a straightforward process (Chapter 2). This is particularly true in several developing countries, which have limited experience of popular participation.

Lack of popular participation, however, exacerbates the risk of new governments dismantling established and on-going programmes. It is much easier for a new mayor to set up his/her own personal agenda if there are no pressures from different sections of the population. Therefore, healthy city projects which have not secured a sound popular basis run a greater risk of being manipulated or even dismantled by an influential politician.

This book argues that popular participation may be the ultimate element which leads to, and supports, sustainability in healthy city projects. Therefore, efforts should be made to support participation as widely as possible in each project. When local communities find a real stake in the project, they will put pressure on any forthcoming mayor to continue it. Popular participation may even guarantee the sustainability of healthy cities beyond the project, an issue which will be analysed next.

FROM HEALTHY CITY PROJECTS TO HEALTHY CITIES BEYOND PROJECTS

This final section briefly discusses whether the Healthy City Project needs to exist indefinitely. The city of Campinas is used as an example to illustrate the discussion. The Campinas Healthy City Project experienced difficulties, which started in 1996 with the death of the mayor who initiated this Project. He died before the completion of his term in office and the deputy mayor, who took his place, did not show the same enthusiasm regarding the Healthy City Project which lost considerable momentum thereafter. At the end of 1996 there were municipal elections, and a candidate from an opposition party won. A new mayor took office in 1997, and has not supported the Healthy City Project.

As noted in Chapter 3, the Campinas Project chose to concentrate action in São Marcos, a low income region of the city. Therefore, considering the changes in office, what happened with the São Marcos initiative? Clearly there has not been political top-down support after the death of the mayor. However, work already implemented in São Marcos, based on strong popular participation (Chapter 3), was sufficient to motivate the local population to fight for its continuation. The actions of such local groups have been backed by technical staff of the local government who worked for the establishment of the São Marcos initiative – the motivation of such staff grew to a point of resisting the demise of the Healthy City Project even without direct support from the mayor. In short, the São Marcos initiative has been pushed forward. The Campinas Healthy City Project may not exist anymore under such a name or label. However, the actions which were established under its umbrella have lived beyond the Project itself.

The above anecdote is a small illustration of the fact that the sustainability of healthy cities should not necessarily mean the long-term survival of the Project. As noted in Chapter 5, although Healthy City Projects is a WHO initiative, its sustainability should not be understood through the narrow approach usually adopted by international agencies, ie that a programme or project should continue to survive, as a programme or project, after the departure of the implementing agency. The Healthy City Project has been implemented in cities and towns which need a systemic change in their approach to urban development and health, in order to improve the well-being of the citizens. At the initial stages, the project implements a system (office, task forces, committees, plans of action, etc) clearly distinguishable from the local/existing system of governance. However, as time goes by, it is expected that both systems blend into each other. Therefore, the aim is not indefinitely to maintain the Healthy City Project's institutional organization, plans of action and the like; but to move from such a situation to the underpinnings of daily public policy. At this point, the project as such may have terminated, but healthy cities will remain alive.

References

Ashton, J (ed) (1992) *Healthy Cities* Open University Press, Buckingham, UK.
Ashton, J and Seymour, H (1988) *The New Public Health: The Liverpool Experience* Open University Press, Milton Keynes, UK.
Atkinson, A (1994) 'Introduction – The Contribution of Cities to Sustainability' *Third World Planning Review* 16(2), pp97–101.
Atkinson, S (1996) 'Applications of Social Research in Urban Health' in Atkinson, S, Songsore, J and Werna, E (eds) *Urban Health Research in Developing Countries: Implications for Policy* CAB International, Wallingford, UK.
Barker, C (1996) *The Health Care Policy Process* Sage, UK.
Barker, C and Green, A (1996) 'Opening the Debate on DALYs' *Health Policy and Planning* 11(2), pp179–183.
Barten, F (1996) *Healthy City Project Managua – Nicaragua: Report of a 2nd visit* Consultancy report for the World Health Organization, April–May 1996.
Baum, F (1993a) 'Noarlunga Healthy Cities Pilot Project: The Contribution of Research and Evaluation' in Davies, J K and Kelly, M P *Healthy Cities: Research and Practice* Routledge, London, UK.
Baum, F (1993b) 'Healthy Cities and Change: Social Movement or Bureaucratic Tool?' *Health Promotion International* 8(1), pp266–285.
Bhatti, M (1988) 'From Consumers to Prosumers: Housing for a Sustainable Future' *Housing Studies* April 8(2), pp98–108.
BKH (Bongaerts, Kuyper and Huiswaard Consulting Engineers) (1989) *Third Chittagong Water Supply and Sanitation Project – Feasibility Study – Final Report: Annexes* October.
BKH (Bongaerts, Kuyper and Huiswaard Consulting Engineers) (1990) *Third Chittagong Water Supply and Sanitation Project – Feasibility Study – Final Report* July.

Blankers, A (1993) *Accra Healthy Cities Project/Urban Primary Health Care – One Year After its Initiation* Research Report, Faculty of Health Sciences, University of Limburg, The Netherlands.

BMA (Bangkok Metropolitan Authority) (1994) *Pilot Project: Healthy Cities* unpublished monograph, Bangkok Metropolitan Administration.

Briggs, D, Corvalan, C and Nurimen, M (eds) (1995) *Linkage Methods for Environment and Health Analysis* WHO/EHG/95.26, WHO, Geneva, Switzerland.

Brugman, J (1994) 'Who Can Deliver Sustainability? Municipal Reform and the Sustainable Development Mandate' *Third World Planning Review* 16(2), pp129–145.

Cairncross, S, Periès, H and Cutts, F (1997) 'Vertical Health Programmes' *The Lancet* 349, pp20–23.

CCC–WHO (Chittagong City Corporation and World Health Organization) (1993) *Chittagong Healthy Cities Project – Health for All – All for Health* CCC/WHO, November.

Choguill, C (ed) (1996) 'Special Issue on Sustainable Development' *Habitat International* 20(3).

Collin, J F (1992) *Guide Notes for the Healthy Cities Indicators* WHO, Regional Office for Europe, Copenhagen, Denmark.

Corvalan, C, Nurminen, M and Pastides, H (eds) (1997) *Linkage Methods for Environment and Health Analysis: Technical Guidelines* WHO/EHG/97.11, WHO, Geneva, Switzerland.

Davey, K (1992) *Central Local Relations* The Institutional Framework of Urban Management Working Paper No. 5, Development Administration Group, University of Birmingham.

Davies, J K and Kelly, M P (1993) *Healthy Cities – Research and Practice* Routledge, London, UK.

Devas, N and Rakodi, C (eds) (1993) *Managing Fast Growing Cities – New Approaches to Urban Planning and Management in the Developing World* Longman Scientific & Technical, Harlow, UK.

Doll, R (1992) 'Health and the Environment in the 1990s' *Am J Public Health* vol 82, pp933–941.

Draper, R, Curtice, L, Hooper, J and Goumans, M (1993) *WHO Healthy Cities Project: Review of the First Five Years (1987–1992) – A*

Working Tool and a Reference Framework for Evaluating the Project WHO, Regional Office for Europe, Copenhagen, Denmark.

Editorial (1991) 'What's New in Public Health?' *The Lancet* 337, pp1381–1383.

Editorial (1992) 'Earth Matters' *The Lancet* 339, pp1325–1326.

Editorial (1996) 'Greening our Health' *The Lancet* 348, pp139.

Elzinger, A (1981) *Evaluating the Evaluation Game: On the Methods of Project Evaluation, with Special Reference to Development Co-operation* SAREC, Stockholm.

Epstein, P (1992) 'Health and Environment' *The Lancet* 340, pp1030–1031.

Feuerstein, M T (1986) *Partners in Evaluation: Evaluating Development and Community Programme with Participants* Macmillan, London, UK.

Goldstein, G and Kickbusch, I (1996) 'A Healthy City is a Better City' *World Health* 1, pp4–6.

Gordon, L (1990) 'Who will Manage the Environment?' *Am J Public Health* 80, pp904–905.

Gordon, L (1991) 'Reaching the Environmental Health Objectives' Editorial, *Journal of Public Health and Policy* 12, pp5–9.

Gordon, L (1992) 'Does Public Health Still Include Environmental Health and Protection?' Editorial, *Journal of Public Health and Policy* 13, pp407–411.

Green, A (1992) *Introduction to Health Planning in Developing Countries* Oxford University Press, UK.

Hardoy, J E, Mitlin, D and Satterthwaite, D (1992) *Environmental Problems in Third World Cities* Earthscan, London, UK.

Harpham, T (1997) *Quetta Healthy City Project, Pakistan: Report of a Visit* WHO consultant's report, May 1997.

Harpham, T and Blue, I (1995) *Fayoum Healthy City Project, Egypt: Start-up Phase* WHO consultants' report, May/June 1995.

Harpham, T and Werna, E (1996a) 'The Idea of Healthy Cities and its Application' in Pugh, C (ed) *Sustainability, the Environment and Urbanization* Earthscan, London.

Harpham, T and Werna, E (1996b) 'Sustainable Urban Health in Developing Countries' *Habitat International* 20(3), pp421–429.

Harris, N (ed) (1992) *Cities in the 1990s – The Challenge for Developing Countries* University College London Press, London, UK.

Harrison, T (1996) *Healthy Cities and Local Agenda 21: The Problem of Evaluating Initiatives and Progress Towards Sustainable Urban Development and Health* Paper presented at the ESRC seminar on Evaluating Urban Policy, University of the West of England, UK 16 December 1996.

Hunt, S M (1993) 'The Relationship between Research and Policy: Translating Knowledge into Action' in Davies, J K and Kelly, M P (eds) *Healthy Cities: Research and Practice* Routledge, London, UK.

Kickbusch, I (1986) 'Issues in Health Promotion' *Health Promotion* 1, pp437–442.

Kilburn, K (1995) 'The Environmental Health Dilemma: Summarising for the Future' *Archives of Environmental Health* 50, pp262–263.

de Leeuw, E and Goumans, M (1993) *Current Research and Evaluation on Healthy Cities Programmes – A Focus on Community Research Priorities and the Producers and Users of this Research* Paper presented at the International Healthy Cities and Communities Conference, San Francisco, USA December 1993.

Leitman, J (1994) 'The World Bank and the Brown Agenda – Evolution of a Concept' *Third World Planning Review* 16(2), pp116–128.

Lotti, M (1991) 'Health and the Environment' *British Journal of Industrial Medicine* 48, pp433–436.

McDonald, T, Treser, C and Hatlen J (1994) 'Development of an Environmental Health Addendum to the Assessment Protocol for Excellence in Public Health' *Journal of Public Health Policy* 15, pp203–217.

Meadows, D H, Meadows, D L, Rangers, J and Behrens III, W (1974) *The Limits to Growth* Pan Books, London, UK.

Mitlin, D (1992) 'Sustainable Development: A Guide to the Literature' *Environment and Urbanization* 4(1), pp111–124.

Mooney, G and Creese, A (1993) 'Priority Setting for Health Service Efficiency: the Role of Measurement of Burden of Illness' in Jamison, D T, Mosely, W H, Measham, A R and Bobadilla, J L (eds) *Disease Control Priorities in Developing Countries* Published for the World Bank, Oxford University Press, New York, USA.

Mullen, P, Evans, D, Forster, J et al (1995) 'Settings as an Important Dimension in Health Education/Promotion Policy, Programs and Research' *Health Education Quarterly* 22, pp329–345.

Murray, C J L (1994) 'Quantifying the Burden of Disease: the Technical Basis for Disability Adjusted Life Year' *Bulletin of the World Health Organization* 72, pp429–445.

ODA (Overseas Development Administration) (1995) *A Guide to Appraisal, Design, Monitoring, Management and Impact Assessment of Health and Population Projects* ODA, London, UK.

Petersen, A (1996) 'The "Healthy" City, Expertise, and the Regulation of Space' *Health and Place* 2(3), pp157–165.

Rossi-Espagnet, A, Goldstein, G B and Tabibzadeh, T (1991) 'Urbanization and Health in Developing Countries: a Challenge for Health for All' *World Health Statistics Quarterly* 44(1), pp186–245.

Sachs, I (1979) 'Ecodevelopment: a Definition' *Ambio* VIII (2/3).

Schrettenbrunner, A and Harpham, T (1993) 'A Different Approach to Evaluating PHC Projects in Developing Countries; How Acceptable is it to Aid Agencies?' *Health Policy and Planning* 8(2), pp128–135.

Schumaker, EF (1973) *Small is Beautiful – A Study of Economics as if People Mattered* Abacus, London, UK.

Serageldin, I and Cohen, M A (eds) (1994) *The Human Face of the Urban Environment* A Report to the Development Community on the Second Annual Conference on Environmentally Sustainable Development, Washington DC September 19–23, Environmentally Sustainable Development Proceedings Series No 5.

Smithies, J and Adams, L (1993) 'Walking the Tightrope: Issues in Evaluation and Community Participation for Health for All' in Davies, J K and Kelly, M P *Healthy Cities: Research and Practice* Routledge, London, UK.

Stoker, G (1990) 'Regulation Theory, Local Government and the Transition from Fordism' in King, D S and Pierre, J (eds), *Challenges to Local Government* Sage, London, UK pp242–264.

Stren, R, White, R and Whitney, J (1992) *Sustainable Cities – Urbanization and the Environment in International Perspective* Westview Press, Boulder, USA.

Tarimo, E and Webster, E G (1994) *Primary Health Care Concepts and Challenges in a Changing World* SHS Paper No 7, WHO/SHS/CC/94.2, World Health Organization, Geneva, Switzerland.

Tsouros, A (ed) (1990) *World Health Organization's Healthy City Project: A Project Becomes a Movement (A Review of Progress 1987 to 1990)* Sogess, Milan, Italy.

UNCHS (United Nations Centre for Human Settlements) (1990) *El Pueblo, Los Asentamientos, El Medio Ambiente y El Desarrollo – Mejorar el Entorno de Vida para un Futuro Sostenible* UNCHS, Nairobi.

UNCHS (United Nations Centre for Human Settlements) (1996) *An Urbanizing World. Global Report on Human Settlements* Oxford University Press, Oxford, UK.

UNCHS–UNEP (United Nations Centre for Human Settlements and United Nations Environment Programme) (1996) *Implementing the Urban Environment Agenda*, A Paper Prepared for the Global Meeting of Cities and International Programmes held during the Habitat II Conference, Istanbul, Turkey 1 June 1996.

UNCHS–UNEP (United Nations Centre for Human Settlements and United Nations Environment Programme) (1997) *Implementing the Urban Environment Agenda – Vol 1* Environmental Planning and Management (EPM) Source Book, UNCHS–UNEP, Nairobi, Kenya.

Walker, B (1994) 'Impediments to the Implementation of Environmental Policy' *Journal of Public Health Policy* 15, pp186–202.

Walt, G (1994) *Health Policy: An Introduction to Process and Power* Witwatersrand University Press, Johannesburg, South Africa and Zed Books, London, UK.

Ward, B and Dubos, R (1972) *Only One Earth – Care and Maintenance of a Small Planet* Penguin, London, UK.

Werna, E (1994) *Urban Management, Provision of Health-related Services and the Healthy City Project in Chittagong, Bangladesh* Research Report, Urban Health Programme, London School of Hygiene and Tropical Medicine.

Werna, E (1995a) *The Chittagong Healthy City Project: Follow-up Analysis One Year After Its Initiation* Research Report, Urban Health Programme, London School of Hygiene and Tropical Medicine.

Werna, E (1995b) *Quetta Healthy City Programme, Pakistan – Start-up phase* Consultancy Report for WHO, August.

Werna, E (1995c) 'The Management of Urban Development or the Development of Urban Management? Problems and Premises of an Elusive Concept' *Cities* 12(5), pp353–359.

Werna, E (1995d) 'Urban Management and Intra-urban Differentials in São Paulo' *Habitat International* 19(1), pp123–138.

Werna, E (1995e) *The Cox's Bazar Healthy Town Plan of Action* Consultancy Report for WHO, April.

Werna, E (1996a) *Chittagong Healthy City Programme, Bangladesh – Review of Progress, August–September 1996* Consultancy Report for WHO, October.

Werna, E (1996b) *Quetta Healthy City Programme, Pakistan – Review of the Start-up Phase and Preparation of the Organisation Phase* Consultancy Report for WHO, May.

Werna, E (1996c) 'United Nation's Agencies' Urban Policies and Health' in Atkinson, S, Songsore, J and Werna, E (eds), *Urban Health Research: Implications for Policy* CAB International, Wallingford, UK pp11–30.

Werna, E (1997) *Fayoum Healthy City Programme, Egypt: Review of Progress* WHO consultant's report, May 1997.

Werna, E and Harpham, T (1995) 'The Evaluation of Healthy City Projects in Developing Countries' *Habitat International* 19(4), pp629–641.

Werna, E, Blue, I and Harpham, T (1996) 'The Changing Agenda for Urban Health' in Cohen, M A, Ruble, B A and Tulchin, J S and Garland, A M (eds) *Preparing for the Urban Future: Global Pressures and Local Forces* Woodrow Wilson Centre Press, Washington DC, USA pp200–222.

White, R R (1994) 'Strategic Decisions for Sustainable Urban Development in the Third World' *Third World Planning Review* 16(2), pp103–116.

WHO (1981) *Development of Indicators for Monitoring Progress Towards Health for All by the Year 2000* Health for All Series No 4, WHO, Copenhagen, Denmark.

WHO (1988) *Improving Urban Health: Guidelines for Rapid Appraisal to Assess Community Health Needs, a Focus on Health Improvements for Low-Income Areas* WHO/SHS/NHP/88.4, WHO, Geneva, Switzerland.

WHO (1990) *Working Group on Indicators of Healthy Cities, Summary Report* WHO, Copenhagen, Denmark.

WHO (1991) *City Networks for Health* Technical Discussion Paper, May.

WHO (1992) *Twenty Steps for Developing a Healthy Cities Project* First edition WHO, Regional Office for Europe, Copenhagen, Denmark.

WHO (1993) *The Urban Health Crisis – Strategies for Health for All in the Face of Rapid Urbanization* WHO, Geneva, Switzerland.

WHO (1995a) *Building a Healthy City: A Practitioners Guide – a Step-by-Step Approach to Implementing Healthy City Projects in Low-Income Countries* WHO, Geneva, Switzerland.

WHO (1995b) *WHO Healthy Cities: A Programme Framework* WHO, Geneva, Switzerland.

WHO (1995c) *A Review of the Operation and Future Development of the WHO Healthy Cities Programme* WHO, Geneva, Switzerland.

WHO (1995d) *Twenty Steps for Developing a Healthy Cities Project* Second edition, WHO, Regional Office for Europe, Copenhagen, Denmark.

WHO (1996a) *New Challenges for Public Health: Report of an Inter-regional Meeting* WHO, Geneva, Switzerland.

WHO (1996b) *Investing in Health Research and Development* Oxford University Press, Oxford, UK.

WHO (1996c) *Creating Healthy Cities in the 21st Century* WHO, Geneva, Switzerland.

WHO (1996d) *Environmental Health Indicators* Draft report, WHO, Geneva, Switzerland.

WHO (1996e) *Think and Act Globally and Intersectorally to Protect National Health* WHO, Geneva, Switzerland.

WHO (1997a) *WHO Healthy Cities Technical Symposium on Evaluation* WHO, Copenhagen, Denmark.

WHO (1997b) *Intersectoral Action for Health: A Cornerstone for Health for All in the 21st Century* Report of the International Conference held in Halifax, Canada, 20-23 April 1997.

Wilkinson, R G (1996) *Unhealthy Societies: the Afflictions of Inequality* Routledge, London, UK.

World Bank (1991) *Urban Policy and Economic Development – An Agenda for the 1990s* World Bank Policy Paper, World Bank, Washington DC, US.

World Bank (1993) *World Development Report: Investing in Health* Oxford University Press, Oxford, UK.

World Resources Institute (1996) *The Urban Environment 1996–1997* A Joint Publication of the World Resources Institute, the United Nations Environment Programme, the United Nations Development Programme, and the World Bank, Oxford University Press, Oxford, UK.

Index

Page numbers in **bold** refer to boxes, tables and figures

Accra, Ghana 26, **28–9**, 83
advocacy 8, 14, 17–18, 20
agencies
  aid 1, 126–7
  donor 91
  international 51, 87, 91
  public 129–30
Agenda 21 3, 6–7
agriculture 9
alienation 53, 54
Alma Ata Conference 3, 5–6, 19
American Public Health Association 13
assessments 27, 75
Australia 89–90
awareness raising **29**, 42, 45, 48, 72, 130

Bangkok, Thailand **116–18**
Bangladesh 60 *see also* Chittagong
Brazil 26, **28–9**, 64, **81–3**, **84**, 133
Bristol 101–3
bureaucracy 36, 37
business 51, 62

Campinas, Brazil 26, 64, **81–3**, 133
capacity building 8, 24, 93, **96–7**, 111
Chittagong, Bangladesh
  awareness raising 45
  community participation 48–9
  funding 46
  government involvement **38–9**, 40, 41, 119–20
  healthy city project 21–2, 25, **30**, **35–6**, 41, 52, 120–1
  local authority involvement 37, 38, 44, 130

NGOs in 49–50
priority setting **84**
private sector in 51
steering committee **23**
sustainability of projects **112–15**
urban development in 108
City Health Plan 22, 27–30, 50, 52, 66–7, 69, 72
City Summit *see* Habitat II
community participation
  in City Health Plan **77–9**
  in evaluation 89–90, 98, 99
  in identifying problems 70–1
  indicators of 93, **97**
  in information gathering 64, 68
  and local authorities 132
  in priority setting 68, 69, 84, 125
  in projects 24, 27, 28, 48–9, 61, 131–2
co-ordination council *see* steering committee
cost benefit analysis 100
cottage industry 9, 75
crime 2, 54

Dakar, Senegal 128
data
  analysis 54–5
  demographic 57
  qualitative 62–4, **65**, 87
  quality of 68
  quantitative 62–4, **65**, 87
  see also information
disability-adjusted life years (DALYs) 57–9
disease
  analysis 57–9

burden 11, 57–9, 71, 86–7
  in cities 2, 5–6, 9
  prevention 8, 108–9
  and public health 8
dose-response function 54

Earth Summit *see* Rio Summit
ecological analysis 54
economic issues 53, 59
education
  environmental 75
  for health **28**, 75, 76
  of workers 75
Egypt **77–9**
empowerment 64
England 3, 7–8
environment
  health issues 9, 12–14, 32, 53–5
  sustainability 105
  in urban development 6–7, 12, 105
environmental health 6, 12–14, 32–3
envisioning 31
epidemiological surveys 27, 54, 93
equity 64, 76 *see also* inequality
establishing projects 21–51
Europe 4–5, 19, 73–4
evaluation 66, 86–103
exposure indicators **94–5**
exposures 54

Fayoum, Egypt **77–9**
food safety 9, 75
forums 49
funding
  external 43, 51, 111, **114–15**, **118**, 126–7
  indicators **96**
  international 87, 91, 111, **114–15**, 126–7
  NGOs 50
  projects 41, 46–7, 51, 53

geographical information systems (GIS) 54–5
Ghana 26, **28–9**, 83
Glasgow, Scotland 42
government
  health policy 31–4
  involvement in projects 38–41, 119–20
  local *see* local authorities
  responsibilities 7, 8, 12–15, **29**, 32
guidelines 21, 22–33, 55–6, 68–9

Habitat II 3, 7, 14, 16, 19
HEADLAMP method 55
health burden *see* disease
health care
  curative 8, 76, 107
  preventive 5, 6, 8, 75, 76
  primary 4, 5–6, 10
  vertical approach 108–9
Health for All Strategy 4, **5**, 19, 102
Health of Towns Association 7–8
Health People 2000 13
health sector
  and environmental health 12–14
  in intersectoral collaboration 10–12
  responsibilities 6–7, 12–14, 33–4
  role in projects 31–4, 40–1
  and the WHO 130–31
health services
  in cities 5–6
  and health 8, 10, 16, 106–7
  improving 76
  planning 57
  provision 8, 61
Health-Culture 7, 19
Healthy Cities and Sustainable Cities 59–60
holistic approach
  to health issues 4, 10, 18, 58
  to projects 51, 52, 124
  to urban development 92, 93
horizontal approach *see* intersectoral collaboration
housing 2, 9, 11, 32, 50

Ibadan, Nigeria 59–60, 128–9
identity 31
illiteracy 48, 69, 71
impact indicators 87, 88, 90–98
implementation 35, 52–85
India 128
indicators 87, 90–99
industry
  health issues 9, 11
  partnerships 75

145

and projects 62
small-scale 9, 75
worker participation 75
inequality 53, 54 *see also* equity
information
analysis 20
communication 48
gathering 55–6, 62–6, 68, 70, 83
organization of **56**
and policymaking 67–8, 83
prioritising 70
sources of 62
see also data
insecurity 2, 53, 54
institutional organization 22–6, 27, 36–40, 60, **113–14**
integrated approach *see* holistic approach; intersectoral collaboration
international agencies 51, 87
international aid 87, 91, 111, **114–15**, 126–7
international indicators 98–9
international initiatives 74, 127–9
intersectoral collaboration
case studies **23**, **113**, **116–7**
in City Health Plans **28**, 120
in health issues 8, 9–14, 110
in health policy 31–4
in international initiatives 127–9
local authorities 16–18, 36–7, 41, 123–4
in primary health care 10
in priority setting 69, 125
problems 123–4
in public health 9–14
for sustainability 107
in task forces 26
Iran 84
IULA 131

Japan 7, 19
Johannesburg, South Africa **84**, 128

Lahore, Pakistan **28–9**, **84**
Latin America 7, 19
LIFE programme 49, 50
linkages 11, 27, 54–5, 56, 84
Liverpool, England 42, 69

living conditions
health issues 2, 3, 9, 10, 11–12, 14, 16, 18
urban areas 5–6
local action 8, 24, 120
Local Agenda 21 (LA21) 6–7
local authorities
and community participation 132
employees 130
health issues 4, 6–7
health promotion 19–20
inspection procedures 75–6
institutional organization 36–40, 60
international initiatives 74
intersectoral collaboration 16–18, 36–7, 41, 123–4
involvement in projects 44, 46–7
Local Agenda 21 (LA21) 6–7
motivation 129–30
policies 44, 47, 60, 73
in projects 38–40, 130–31
responsibilities 6–7
steering committees 22
and urban development 14–16
vertical approach 123–4
and the WHO 130–31
local indicators 98–9

Madras, India 128
Managua, Nicaragua 83
Mandalay, Myanmar 26
marginalisation 53, 54, 73
market places 75–6
mental illness 2, 9, 57
Mexico 127
monitoring 20, 46, **95–6**
mortality 12, 54, 57
motivation 130
multi-city action plans (MCAPs) 73–4, 111
municipal government *see* local authorities
Municipal Health Plan *see* City Health Plan
Myanmar 26

National Healthy Cities Commission 72–3
networks 24, 61, 72–4, 99, 111, 120–21

Index

New Economics Foundation 100
NGOs 42, 49–50
Nicaragua 83
Nigeria 59–60, 128–9
Noarlunga, Australia 89–90

occupational health 9–10, 11, 75
organization, institutional 22–6, 27, 36–40, 60, **113–14**
Ottawa Charter 3, 4–5, 19
overcrowding 2, 5–6

PAHO 130
Pakistan *see* Lahore; Quetta
partnerships
  community 17, 24, 129
  for health care 76
  in health policy 34
  in projects **29**, **30**, 32, 47–51, 59–60
  service provision 15
  stakeholder 35, 40–1
  in workplaces 75
phases of projects 27–34
pilot projects **80–81**, 91–2
policy (health) 20, 31–4
pollution 2, 9, 11, 32, 75
popular participation 49
population growth 2, 15
poverty 1, 2, 9, **35**, 53–4
primary health care 4, 5–6, 10
priority setting **29**, 66–72, 84, 125
private sector 51
problems
  identifying **29**, 57–8, 66, 70–71, **77–8**, 125
  solving **29**, 66, 71
process indicators 87, 88, 90–98
project approach 123
project office 24–5, 27, 38, 45–7
projects
  communicating **29**, 41–2, 45, 48, 72, 130
  designing 124–5
  establishing 21–53
  funding 41, 46–7, 51, 53
  guidelines 21, 22–33, 55–6, 68–9
  implementing 35, 52–85
  phases 27–34
  pilot **89–81**, 91–2

  prioritising 66–72
  sustainability 111, **112–8**, 133–4
promotion 4
public health
  and environmental health 13
  health care provision 3–4, 7–8, 13
  history 7–8
  improvements 3–4
  intersectoral collaboration 9–14
  responsibility for 3–4, 12–14, 32–3
Public Health Act (1848) 7
public sector 34–5, 130–31

qualitative data 13, 93
quality of life 13
Quetta, Pakistan
  awareness raising 42, 45
  City Health Plan **79–81**
  community participation 48–9
  funding 47
  government involvement 39, 40–1
  healthy city project 21–2, 25–6, **35–6**, 42, 52
  local authority involvement 37, 38, 39–40, 44
  NGOs in 49, 50
  priority setting **79–81**
private sector in 51

rapid appraisal techniques 64, 66
reporting 8, 45, 90
research 8, 13, 67
resources
  external 43, 51, 111, **114–15**, **118**, 126–7
  financial 67, 71
  local 111, **114–15**, **118**
  non-financial 42–3, 67, 71, 111
  pooling 42–3
Rio de Janeiro, Brazil **28–9**, **84**
Rio Summit (1992) 3, 6–7, 14
risk analysis 54
risk assessment 75

safety
  food 9, 75
  at work 9–10, 11, 75
'sanitary idea' 3, 7–8
sanitation 9

147